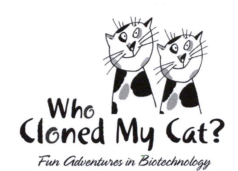

Who Cloned My Cat?

Fun Adventures in Biotechnology

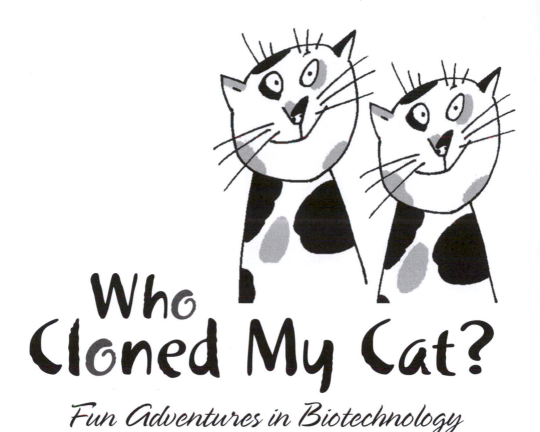

Who Cloned My Cat?

Fun Adventures in Biotechnology

Cartoons by **Manfred Bofinger** and **Ming Fai Chow**

Reinhard Renneberg
Hong Kong University of Science and Technology, Hong Kong

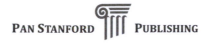
PAN STANFORD PUBLISHING

Published by

Pan Stanford Publishing Pte. Ltd.
Penthouse Level, Suntec Tower 3
8 Temasek Boulevard
Singapore 038988

Email: editorial@panstanford.com
Web: www.panstanford.com

British Library Cataloguing-in-Publication Data
A catalogue record for this book is available from the British Library.

WHO CLONED MY CAT?
Fun Adventures in Biotechnology

Translation from the German language edition:

Katzenklon by Reinhard Renneberg

Copyright © 2011 Spektrum Akademischer Verlag

Spektrum Akademischer Verlag is an imprint of Springer Science+Business Media

ISBN-13 978-981-4267-65-6
ISBN-10 981-4267-65-1

Printed in Singapore.

To Louiza – My Love and Best Friend

Foreword

Chance Favors the Prepared Mind

It's my belief that nobody reads forewords... but my publisher has asked me to write this anyway — to explain a little *why* I'm so fond of teaching, writing, nature and life, and how a German came to be a biotech professor in Hong Kong...

Teaching is one of my obsessions. Maybe it's because I was born — July 2, 1951 — *in* a school. My young parents, Herbert and Ilse, were the only teachers in the small village of Lössen near Merseburg in the former East Germany. They lived on the first floor of the same building where they taught half days on the floor below. My grandparents, owners of a small farm, lived on the other side of the road. So, I grew up with rabbits, pigs, chickens, doves, cows and a horse. And I loved the family's dachshund.

Apparently, the school kids spoiled me. To score points with their beloved teachers — and find an excuse to avoid class — they wheeled me non-stop around the tiny school in a baby buggy. (It's any wonder that I didn't become a racecar driver; in fact, just the opposite happened: out of environmental concerns, I would turn against cars.) My Dad later moved to the small town of Merseburg and worked as a biology teacher, eventually becoming the principal. During our frequent nature walks, my Mom could name all the flowers — very impressive!

I attended the "Ernst Haeckel" High School in Merseburg. Haeckel became an early hero of mine: he was a spirited advocate of Darwin's theory, and during his school years he had amassed a plant collection of almost 10,000 species from the district of Merseburg alone! He later traveled to exotic countries and published beautiful and very popular books on nature and evolution — complete with illustrations based on his own drawings. He was a giant of knowledge. I also tried my hand at drawing nature; my Dad was quite good at it. These days I like sketching cartoons for my students — and Chinese students *love* cartoons...

Unlike most other children, I adored school and admired my teachers. Maybe I was just lucky to have dedicated ones who were full of passion. Today, I try my best to pass on this enthusiasm to my students and readers. *You cannot give the fire of knowledge to others if you yourself do not burn!* and *Science is fun!* are my mottos — together with Louis Pasteur's *Chance favors the prepared mind.*

It was clear to me at an early stage that studying life and nature would be my profession. What could be more interesting? My parents would buy me kits with experiments on chemistry and biology. I joined the Merseburg birdwatchers on excursions, and I still love birds to this day. Later, I chanced upon a copy of *The Double Helix* (1968) by celebrated American molecular biologist James Watson. I had a new hero, and I was soon constructing my own DNA models at home.

For my studies, I wanted to move as far away as possible from East Germany. But this was no simple matter in 1970. The Berlin Wall had been built in 1961 and the Cold War between East and West was simmering. The farthest would have been Beijing, but the Russians, East Germany's allies, had fallen out with the Chinese communists. So, I went to what was then the Soviet Union, to universities in an unknown city named Donetsk and a rather more famous place called Moscow.

Student life was hugely enriching and I traveled the length and breadth of the Soviet Empire, from the Baltic states to Siberia and the Middle East. I discovered wonderful people, breathtaking scenery, and inept economic systems! My teacher at the Soviet Academy of Sciences was Vladimir Konstantinovich Antonov. He impressed me not only with his astonishing knowledge of science but also of poetry and, like most Russians, of music. A true Renaissance man!

Coming home, I joined the Academy of Sciences in East Berlin. I was again fortunate to have a great teacher, and later a valued friend: Frieder Scheller took biosensor research in East Germany to a world-class level. I learned from Frieder to be innovative — and to make the most of every situation.

It was then that I got married to Ilka in Berlin, a chemist I knew from Moscow. We have two sons, Max and Tom.

During those years, my research work alone proved insufficiently fulfilling; I needed to *teach*. A Leipzig publisher Bernd Scheiba convinced me that I should write my first popular science book on biotechnology — quite a challenge, since the main biotech developments were in the West, and there I was in the East. Good Western books were rare; information was hard to come by. But I got lucky again when I met a marvelously talented lady called Darja Suessbier, who could perform small miracles with her art. (We still collaborate today.) And I also came to know the late Manfred Bofinger — a genius cartoonist of his time.

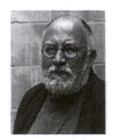

Manfred Bofinger

Yet another lottery win came my way when I was invited to work as a post-doc in the epicenter of biotechnology — Japan. There, I worked day and night, absorbing all the biotech knowledge I possibly could, buying all the terrific illustrated Japanese biotech books and journals around, and enjoying wonderful working relationships with the late Professor Saburo Fukui, Takashi Kakiuchi, Isao Karube and Masuo Aizawa.

All that time, East Germany had remained isolated. But in the Autumn of 1989, I suddenly found myself with my sons Max and Tom tearing down The Wall with our own hands... How surreal to be a part of world history! The Greek philosophers had it right: *panta rhei*. Everything flows.

After unification, I moved to the Western part of the "Fatherland", to Münster, and was immediately appointed Department Head at the Fraunhofer Institute for Chemical and Biosensors. But the allure of exotic lands was more potent. After I was invited to give a talk in Hong Kong, I was so impressed by Asia that I accepted a professorship at the region's most modern technical institution, the Hong Kong University of Science and Technology, HKUST. This paradise of research, education, culture and nature is where I am still. And I've since started two companies.

It was Merlet Braunbeck from Spektrum Akademischer Verlag in Heidelberg who persuaded me to write a book on biotechnology. Every two weeks I was contributing a short popular article called *Biolumne* to a German newspaper, and Merlet came up with the idea of publishing a collection of those articles. But that book was in German, and even the most talented of my new Asian students sadly could not get much out of it...

My collaboration with the cartoonist Manfred Bofinger had begun with an earlier book called *Liebling, du hast die Katze geklont!* (*Honey, you cloned the cat!*). I called him from Hong Kong and said, "Manfred, I'm working on a book about biotechnology, which should be easy to read and funny too. I would like to have some nice illustrations in the book and I already have an idea: Could you draw me a detergent enzyme at work? Maybe as a tiny person with a saw and scissors in its hands, chopping up any substrate it can find?"

"Send me a fax with a sketch!" Manfred grumbled. I did it immediately. A reply was faxed two hours later. The great Bofi, who had illustrated my children's reading and maths books, sent *me* a fax!

It was a pig wearing a suit and a tie, sitting at a table with an alien and saying: "How fascinating! Alkaline protease, you are a fellow omnivore?" (Find the illustration in Chap. 45, *Molecular Laundresses*, p. 96.) That was so him! Bofi had simply ignored my boring idea. Good friends told me: "Well, thank God he didn't listen to you!" I received new illustrations from Bofi every two weeks, and they all turned out to be quite different from my simple sketches. I was completely addicted. Every time his fax arrived felt like Christmas.

Until that terrible moment in 2004. I had been waiting for Bofi's fax for days until I finally heard from his wife Gaby that he had developed agrypnocoma, a serious and debilitating lethargic condition. Unbelievable: he was such a lively and energetic man. Manfred Bofinger died on January 8, 2006. His joy of life, his faith in goodness and his sanity were contagious.

Bofi was irreplaceable, but I had no choice but to look for a new cartoonist. I found him in the *South China Morning Post*: Ming's funny and sharp-witted illustrations were a hit in Hong Kong. After some persistent research, I found his address and we arranged to meet. I presumed that he must be quite old, older than me at least. A fun guy in his thirties showed up — Ming's son? No, it was the master himself!

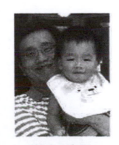

Ming and Son

He was concerned after he saw Bofi's works. "I would never be able to do that!" he said. But Ming found his own style and he was so much fun to work with.

And so, we finally come to my most recent piece of good fortune and the book you now hold in your hands — thanks to a creative and innovative Singapore publisher, Stanford Chong, who earned my trust immediately when I saw the beautiful, educational books he publishes.

But now, dear reader, enough about the author… *Enjoy the book!*

Reinhard Renneberg

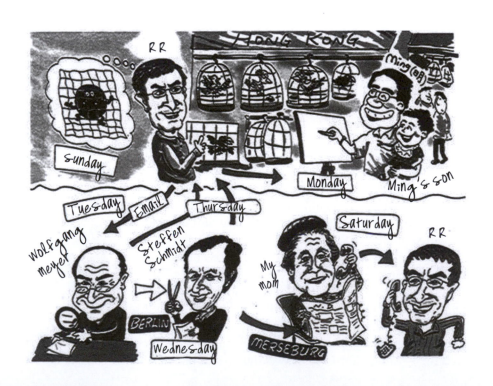

Contents

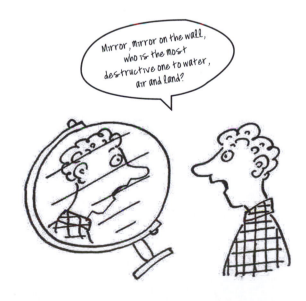

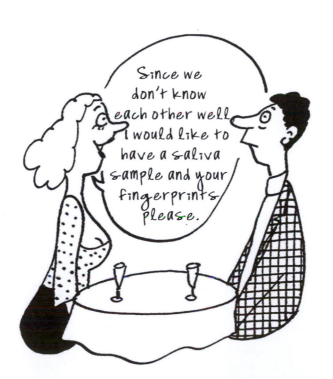

Chapter 1

Will Biotech Banish Wrinkles Forever?

Wipe out your wrinkles with anti-aging creams? I doubt it. We all know that even the best anti-aging products can only smoothen the signs of aging; despite what they claim, they can't work miracles. And then there are the people who use the "B-weapon": Botulinus toxin (Botox), a toxin formed by bacteria that are notorious for food poisoning. Injected under the skin, Botox paralyzes the muscles, and the wrinkles disappear — at least for a while.

At my university, the Hong Kong University of Science and Technology (HKUST), a new substance is in use: it is called Epidermal Growth Factor (EGF). EGF is nothing new — a peptide that stimulates the splitting and regeneration of skin cells. As we age, less EGF is produced. If the EGF can be "fed," cell regeneration will be well underway again.

My colleague, Prof. Wan-Keung Wong, produces this valuable substance genetically using bacteria. EGF, from a bioreactor, has exactly the same structures and effects as the original molecule produced by the human body.

The new substance is now in use in creams in China, but with quite a high price tag: one small tube (20 mg) sets you back about 70 US-dollars in Hong Kong and might last for only two weeks. But after four to six weeks of daily use, your wrinkles will be replaced by regenerated skin cells.

Well, I can personally vouch for this new treatment — I played vain guinea pig and tested it myself. Sure enough: the wrinkles around my eyes were gone after four weeks, even if my frown and laughter lines stubbornly refused to disappear.

So can anything be said scientifically against EGF? It's hard to say for sure what will happen after long-term use — if one tries too hard to rejuvenate oneself. Will the "spoiled" skin age faster if EGF is no longer administered?

Even Europeans, renowned skeptics when it comes to using genetically engineered products, will probably take the plunge — because it really seems to work. Still, there are legitimate concerns that shouldn't be overlooked: What would happen if a beauty fanatic combined EGF with a solarium treatment and it came into contact with skin cancer cells?

Who Cloned My Cat? Fun Adventures in Biotechnology by R. Renneberg
Copyright © 2011 by Pan Stanford Publishing Pte Ltd
www.panstanford.com
978-981-4267-65-6

Worries aside, EGF has made possible at least one medical breakthrough for severe diabetic patients, who often suffer from diabetic foot ulcers or open wounds that will not heal. By using EGF for only eight weeks, a research team in Hong Kong managed to prevent foot amputation, which would otherwise have been unavoidable.

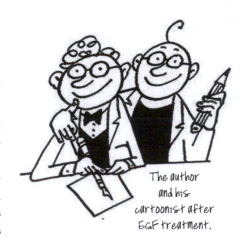

The author and his cartoonist after EGF treatment.

EGF also works wonders for sunburn — although that is not a problem here in China, where having pale skin is a sign of beauty. My students' umbrellas go up the moment the sun comes out, and they giggle at us "long noses" who go to the beach to get a tan or even spend money in tanning salons. Maybe the Chinese really are smarter than us. The dermatologists and the skin cancer statistics certainly prove them right.

In case you're wondering, my wrinkles have all returned now that I've run out of that expensive cream. It looks like I'll have to live with my well-earned lines after all.

My son Tom, the computer nerd, offers the only comfort: "Daddy, I'll get rid of your wrinkles in five minutes for nothing — with Adobe Photoshop®!"

Chapter 2

The Breast Milk of Civilization

There is an old saying: *He who has cares, has liquor also.* Could there be other good reasons for the invention of alcoholic beverages besides Wilhelm Busch's humorous wisdom? Biotechnologists and historians seem to think so.

Living between the Euphrates and Tigris rivers between 6,000 to 8,000 years ago, the Sumerians — who founded the Mesopotamian civilization — had already mastered the art of brewing. So important was the nutritious juice that beer brewers were required to stay at home in times of war.

The Sumerians' successors, the Babylonians, were already choosing between some 20 different kinds of beer. The brewery was an important national interest for them, so much so that their great King Hammurapi proclaimed that a brewer who is found to be watering down their beer should be drowned in their barrels or made to drink themselves to death with their own brew.

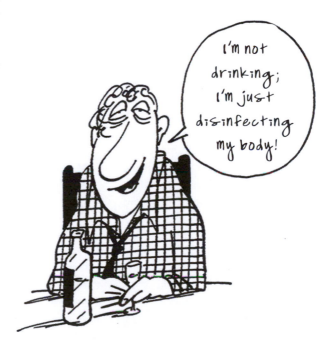

Alcohol (the layman's term for ethanol) is essentially sugar which enzymatically splits up, a product of yeast metabolism, and doesn't really feed other microbes (besides ethanoic acid bacteria) producing vinegar from ethanol. In addition, alcohol damages the cell wall of bacteria.

Who Cloned My Cat? Fun Adventures in Biotechnology by R. Renneberg
Copyright © 2011 by Pan Stanford Publishing Pte Ltd
www.panstanford.com
978-981-4267-65-6

Babylonian beer had a slightly sour taste to it, which was a result of the process of lactic acid fermentation. The lactic acid bacteria made the beer last longer, as most microbes cannot survive in an acidic environment. It was food preservation through fermentation of lactic acid — just like with pickled gherkins, sauerkraut and olives.

In the hot climate of the Middle East, microbial inhibition through fermentation was greatly advantageous, if not crucial. As a result of extensive agriculture, the population grew dramatically. Soon, the paucity of clean drinking water became a problem, as it did in Europe until into the 19th century.

With a lack of canals and poor or non-existent sewage reprocessing, animal and human feces still contaminate drinking water in various places today.

Just five percent of China's water is thought to be "safe" (though here industrial pollution is to blame). Even ritual washing, such as in the Ganges in India, is an issue. Contaminated water can be highly dangerous.

In contrast, fermented products such as beer, wine and vinegar are free from dangerous germs. They could even be used to make moderately contaminated water safe, given that alcohol and organic acids kill potential pathogens.

Napoleon's soldiers used to add red wine to water from an unknown origin. "I am not drinking; I am disinfecting my body!" is a popular joke among those who love to drink — and it is not entirely untrue. Alcohol was the only available analgesic until a hundred years ago. Imagine: brandy as an anesthetic!

So, it was not water that quenched the thirst of our ancestors but beer, wine and vinegar — the "breast milk of civilization." This venerable biotechnology provided stimulating drinks that nurtured civilization and were relatively safe at the same time — a revolutionary technology that we just couldn't help but inherit.

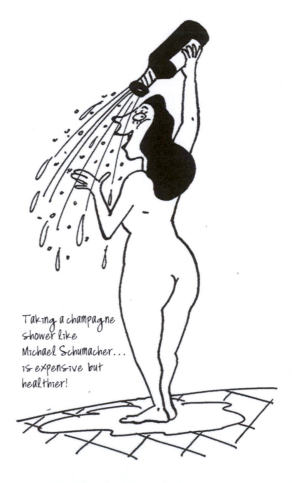

Taking a champagne shower like Michael Schumacher... is expensive but healthier!

Chapter 3

The Little Roaring Mouse

"China had three big triumphs to celebrate in 2003: the first Chinese person in outer space, victory against the SARS virus (Severe Acute Respiratory Syndrome), and participation in the Human Genome Project," rejoiced Prof. Huanming Yang, head of the Beijing Genome Institute.

"To sequence or not to sequence, that is the question!" he bellowed to an enthusiastic Hong Kong crowd. Hong Kong finally had its own genome center.

The target of the Human Genome Project (HGP) was to decipher (meaning determine the chronological base pairs in genetic vectors inside DNA molecules) all human chromosomes. The biggest biological project of all time, it began in October 1990 with a research fund of 3 billion US dollars.

Biotechnologists have been working nonstop on the data ever since in an effort to list all of the roughly 3.4 billion base pairs allocated in the 23 human chromosome pairs. The amount of information could be printed in about 200 telephone books each with over 1,000 pages. The smallest chromosome X (with "a little difference") has around 50 million base pairs, while the biggest has 250 million.

Knowledge gained from the human genome promises to change the biological and medical world dramatically. Around 6,000 diseases have been attributed to one single damaged gene; one misspelling of a genetic word is enough to produce the wrong kind of protein or the wrong amount of it. In complex diseases, such as heart attack, arteriosclerosis, asthma and cancers, dozens of genes may be involved.

On April 14, 2003, the US, Great Britain, Germany, Japan, France and China (Prof. Yang: "as the only developing nation") jointly announced that the complete human genome had been deciphered. China, though, joined the "genome club" as the sixth member only at the end of 1999. The Chinese decoded only one percent of the genome, making them the mouse among the great elephants (USA: 54 percent; Great Britain: 37 percent). Still, they were at least in the club — unlike the Russians!

Who Cloned My Cat? Fun Adventures in Biotechnology by R. Renneberg
Copyright © 2011 by Pan Stanford Publishing Pte Ltd
www.panstanford.com
978-981-4267-65-6

And to whom does the human genome "belong"? Who is the owner of this highly prized patent? Jiang Zemin, then-president of the People's Republic of China, provided an answer: "It belongs to all, it was encoded by all and should be shared among all!"

And that was how the Chinese genome mouse roared like a tiger: *The human genome belongs to everyone; it cannot and should not be patented.* It wasn't only the *Wall Street Journal* that found the Chinese statements unpalatable. The US Centers for Disease Control in Atlanta were in the process of trying to patent the genome of the SARS virus at the time. Of course, the Chinese were outraged. After all, the virus was isolated and classified in Hong Kong.

Those in Hong Kong who pay attention would also have appreciated the additional reasons for the genome elephants' astonishment: ten thousand Chinese students in the US, who are sometimes referred to by US researchers as "Chinese tools," learn diligently from "the master." Most of them return home perfectly skilled. In the meantime the Chinese have decoded the genomes of rice (55,000 genes) and silkworms, and are working hard on chickens and pigs.

The first VIP to arrive in Hong Kong was a pioneer of genome research, Craig Venter, from the US (see Chap. 77, *DNA Gunshots into the Sea*, p. 169 and Chap. 80, *Microbesoft*, p. 177). Venter's privately funded company went head-to-head in delivering the human genome with the state-aided scientists led by Francis Collins. Ultimately, both were chosen as winners by Bill Clinton in 2001. Venter wrote his signature on one of the DNA sequencing machines in the Hong Kong genome laboratory.

The Hong Kong Genome Institute is, according to Venter, one of the finest. Hong Kong has now gained its place on the world map of genome research.

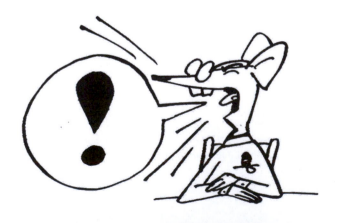

Chapter 4

Expensive and Often Useless

"More than half of the patients who use the most expensive prescriptions don't have any use for them!" Allen Roses, vice president for genetics from the global company Glaxo Smith Kline (GSK), shocked his audience in London with this statement at the end of 2003.

An open secret in the pharmaceutical industry, this was the first time that one of its heads had spoken out about it. Medicines for Alzheimer's disease work for less than one third of patients; those for cancer hardly even work for one quarter of them. Medicines for migraine, osteoporosis and arthritis only help one in two sufferers.[1]

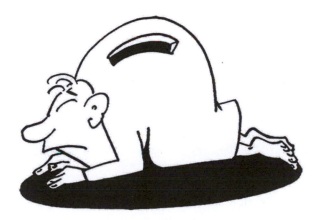

---

[1] The efficiency of medicines is shockingly low (after Allen Roses): Alzheimer's disease: 30 percent; analgesic (pain killer): 80 percent; asthma: 60 percent; arrhythmia: 60 percent; depression (SSRI): 62 percent; diabetes: 57 percent; hepatitis C: 47 percent; incontinence: 40 percent; migraine (acute): 52 percent; migraine (prevention): 50 percent; cancer: 25 percent; rheumatoid arthritis: 50 percent; schizophrenia: 60 percent (see www.independent.co.uk/news/science/glaxo-chief-our-drugs-do-not-work-on-most-patients-575942.html).

Who Cloned My Cat? Fun Adventures in Biotechnology by R. Renneberg
Copyright © 2011 by Pan Stanford Publishing Pte Ltd
www.panstanford.com
978-981-4267-65-6

"The reason for this is the genetic disposition of patients, which interferes with the medicine. The majority of medicines, more than 90 percent, only work for 30 to 50 percent of patients," Roses, a specialist in pharmacogenomics, explained. Mark Levin, head of Millennium Pharmaceuticals, estimates the proportion of unsuitable prescriptions to be from 20 to 40 percent.

That the same medicine works differently for different people is a fact that everyone is aware of. Doctors usually prescribe a certain kind of medicine based on the ailment. If they could take genetic disposition into consideration, it would be a medical revolution. Side-effects would also be reduced.

When genome scientists, for example, identify a group of genes that could be significant in lung cancer, they compare their incidence in a healthy person with those who suffer from the cancer. The difference (polymorphism) between the gene sequences could be a measurement of the possibility of developing the cancer.

It is often only single base pairs that mutate (*single-nucleotide polymorphisms,* SNPs), from A(denine) to G(uanine) or from T(hymine) to C(ytosine). Two million SNPs have already been recorded in databases. They are also known as *snips*.

This information can now be used for diagnostic tests. People with a higher risk of contracting cancer can thus be forewarned. It will also be possible to determine which medicine works best on whom. The beta2AR gene, for example, defines how well an asthma patient reacts to albuterol (the opening of the respiratory tract through lung muscle relaxation). There are, however, four or five different variations (alleles) of this gene. This explains why albuterol doesn't work well in about 25 percent of cases.

Pharmacogenomics could be a double-edged sword for the pharmaceutical industry. The era of "blockbuster drugs for everyone" with billions in profits may well be over. Instead, custom-made pharmaceuticals will be the next big thing — for me "Rennol Super" may turn out to be *my* ideal headache pill.

But won't this lead to medical discrimination? The "off-the-shelf" not-completely-effective medicines for the masses and the "personalized" super-medicines for the wealthy?

Some experts predict that doctors will be able to use genome information in about five years to prescribe tailormade medicines without side-effects — while charging around 500 US dollars per genome analysis. It is expected that by 2040 all doctors will work almost entirely based on their patients' genomes. I will be 89 by then; I am looking forward to it!

Unfortunately, there are others who delight in the idea of having such information: insurance companies, corporate leaders, governments and, of course, the secret services!

Chapter 5

Computers on the Compost Heap

In fits of rage, you might have often wanted to throw your computer into the trash, but this by no means guarantees that it will be properly disposed of — discarded hardware and materials are causing a lot of headaches these days. It seems, however, that the Japanese are once again approaching a solution.

Indeed, customers who receive their bills from the Japanese telephone company NTT DoCoMo are helping the environment (a little): the transparent plastic window on their envelopes begin life not in an oil well but in a cornfield. The window is made of polylactic acid (PLA). Lactate is a salt of lactic acid, well known from sore muscles (see Chap. 12, *"Irasshaimase, Baioteku"*, p. 25) and yogurt advertisements.

In polylactate, lactate is polymerized into one long chain. It is obtained from glucose by microbial fermentation of cornstarch. Since 2002, a plant in Nebraska, USA, has been producing 140,000 tons of PLA each year, sold under the delightful name "NatureWorks™ PLA." A Japanese company has used it to create, for example, thin transparent plastic sheets. Ten kernels of corn are needed for one A4 sheet.

The bioplastic material is a sensation in Japan. The Japanese have always had to play a leading role in biotechnology. Limited resources — raw materials as well as space for waste disposal — aggravate the problems and force them to innovate. Every year, 15 million tons of kerosene are imported into Japan and tens of thousands of marine creatures around the Japanese islands perish as a direct result of non-biodegradable plastic waste.

Japanese industry is doing its bit too. The automobile giant Toyota announced the use of PLA for spare tire covers and floor mats, while Sanyo launched a biodegradable CD called MildDisc made from PLA. The computer company Fujitsu even plans to sell a "veggie notebook" that has a biodegradable housing!

Only the new material's thermal sensitivity and the price are getting in the way. "It won't have any problem with ice cold cola, but PLA turns soft at 60°C — and who would want to hold a hot melting teacup in their hands?" says Noboyuki

Who Cloned My Cat? Fun Adventures in Biotechnology by R. Renneberg
Copyright © 2011 by Pan Stanford Publishing Pte Ltd
www.panstanford.com
978-981-4267-65-6

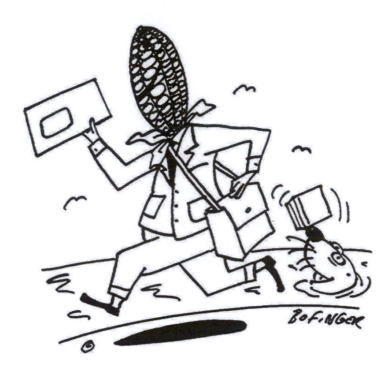

Kawashima of Mitsui Chemicals Ltd. "Of course, we will solve these technical problems!" Biodegradable teabags and tableware are on their way.

But one kilogram of bioplastic for ¥500 is still more than three times more expensive than the kerosene equivalent. Things might change as soon as PLA products go into mass production.

If all plastic waste degraded gracefully one day in the future, that would be a huge biotechnological success story, turning a one-way road (raw material–product–waste) into a succession of natural cycles.

PLA has long been used in the medical world, for example, as self-dissolving threads and even as bone screws. In plastic surgery, PLA is being used as a hydrogel and — needless to say — is a big seller in the anti-aging business. A PLA-based product called New-Fill® is injected especially below deep wrinkles. After four to six weeks a natural rebuilding of the skin volume will take place, and wrinkles and deformations can be reduced. This effect should last (unlike the aforementioned Botox; see Chap. 1, *Will Biotech Banish Wrinkles Forever?* p. 1) for two years or more. Worldwide, around 100,000 patients have been treated with this method.

So if you're looking for gift ideas, treat yourself and your environment — and do without your frown lines for the next couple of years.

Chapter 6

Hanging on to Hangovers

There are countless remedies for a hangover after that rowdy office party: drinking bucket loads (of water, that is) to overcome the dehydration, compensating for the loss of minerals with *rollmops* (pickled herring) and pickled gherkins, or chewing coffee beans (see Chap. 58, *Praising Ginger*, p. 127). The latest insider's tip: fructose. Take a whole load of fruit sugar before going to bed or the next morning, along with plenty of water. Others favor vitamin B_6. I have had good results with both methods.

People with fructose intolerance be warned though: an overdose could be deadly. Ingesting fructose and vitamins from honey and marmalade during breakfast is the safe way to do it — or, of course, eating lots of fresh fruit. And there's an even easier way: by giving your liver enzymes less work to do (through ethanol).

The biochemical cause for hangovers remains a mystery, even though it could make a millionaire out of the founder of an anti-hangover pill.

Canadian scientists have come up with a novel explanation: when you get the common cold, it is the cytokine produced by your white blood cells that is responsible for headaches and feelings of nausea and dizziness. White blood cells are also stimulated by certain ingredients in alcoholic beverages, known as *congemeres*. Dark alcoholic drinks contain more of them. The worst hangovers happen after drinking brandy, followed by cheap red wine, rum, whiskey, white wine, gin, vodka, and finally pure ethanol. Since congemeres are quickly broken down by the body, the effects usually don't last longer than a day.

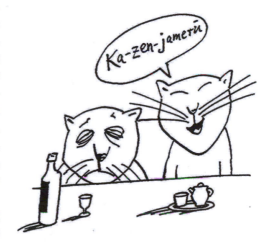

Another miracle cure emerging from the latest US research is cactus

Who Cloned My Cat? Fun Adventures in Biotechnology by R. Renneberg
Copyright © 2011 by Pan Stanford Publishing Pte Ltd
www.panstanford.com
978-981-4267-65-6

extract, which is purported to reduce the effects of a hangover and at the same time lower the concentration of the indicators (C-reactive proteins, CRP) of inflammatory processes. So, a hangover is like inflammation?

That seems plausible, but there are also other interpretations. Many scientists say that it is not congemere that causes hangovers but acetaldehyde, which is produced in the liver by the enzyme alcohol dehydrogenase in the process of breaking down ethanol. Acetaldehyde is later broken down by the enzyme into harmless acetic acid.

My Asian colleagues here in Hong Kong are often amazed at how their liver enzymes are — by nature — not as effective as my *"made in Germany"* ones. Well, mine have also spent five years training in the various countries in the former Soviet Union. Many Chinese and Japanese become merry rather quickly (very economical!) and it can be highly amusing. Their heads turn bright red, and they can have a bad hangover after a relatively small amount of booze. One morning after a *sake* party, one of my Japanese colleagues pointed to my forehead and asked politely, "Ka-zen-ja-meru?" (*Katzenjammer*, German for hangover).

Whether congemeres, cytokines or acetaldehyde is responsible, biochemistry alone is not enough to explain our greatly varied reactions to alcohol consumption. One US study with more than 1,100 participants proved the point: about a quarter didn't suffer a hangover despite excessive drinking. The survey suggested that factors such as guilt, anger, depression and misfortune had a greater influence on the participants' aching heads than how much they drink.

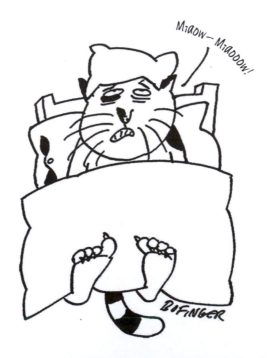

Chapter 7

How Fidel Saved US Biotech

"HFCS" can often be found written on low-calorie drinks; it stands for high fructose corn syrup. HFCS was one of the first modern biotechnology products to be accepted by consumers as a consumer food.

The world's consumption of sugar continues to increase, while sugar cane and sugar beets have not changed their high demands for soil and favorable climatic conditions. But sugar can be extracted from amylases starch (Latin: *amylum*), the natural storage product in plants, as glucose.

Plants with a high starch content (such as potatoes, grain, cassava, and sweet potatoes) are more economical and easy to store, and their cultivation is widespread. Special enzymes (amylases) break down starch into glucose, but this only has three quarters of the sweetness of cane or beet sugar (sucrose), and hence comparatively larger quantities are required.

On the other hand, fruit sugar (fructose) outdoes the sweetness of sucrose by 80 percent, which makes it twice as sweet as glucose. Ingenious: doubling the sweetness by chemical conversion of glucose into fructose — just using enzymes. And at the same time you get a low-calorie sweetener in the bargain (see Chap. 11, *Aspartame: Nothing but Sweetness*, p. 23).

Glucose isomerase (GI) was discovered in 1957, and it has been used since 1967 by the Clinton Corn Processing Company (CCPC) in the USA to produce fructose syrup. Initially, the syrup contained only 15 percent fructose. It didn't take long until they realized that the GI-process can only be cost effective if the expensive enzymes can be used more than once. But how do you make an enzyme re-usable? Answer: it has to be "immobilized" without limiting its activity.

A walk through the Hong Kong bird market demonstrates the concept (see Chap. 21, *Biochemical Bird Market*, p. 45): here we find beautiful Chinese nightingales, confined in gorgeous, but small, wooden cages. Singing contentedly, the hapless birds have little space to move around, and they feed and excrete in the same place — seemingly without thought of escape. They are quite like the residents of Hong Kong...

Who Cloned My Cat? Fun Adventures in Biotechnology **by R. Renneberg**
Copyright © 2011 by Pan Stanford Publishing Pte Ltd
www.panstanford.com
978-981-4267-65-6

By the same token, enzyme molecules can be "locked" in polymer cages. In 1968, CCPC introduced a discontinuous fructose production method using immobilized enzymes that yielded 42 percent fructose. Finally, in 1972, they succeeded in developing a continuous process.

Still, the price of sugar was about 15–20 US cents per kilogram in the 1960s, and the production of fructose syrup was more costly. The skeptics were soon predicting the demise of the sweet, new biotechnology — but a little too hastily as it turned out.

By November 1974, sugar prices had climbed to US$1.25 per kilogram. Cuba, the original sugar supplier to the Western world, had decided to align itself politically and economically with the Soviet Union.

After the Bay of Pigs debacle, sugar cane plantations in the Philippines were expected to help resolve the issue, but there were teething problems. And, almost overnight, the enzyme process started to look very attractive.

By the time the price had dropped again to 15 cents per kilogram at the end of 1976, the new production method was already well established, and fructose syrup was being produced at a lower cost than that of sucrose. Meanwhile, the disappointment of unfulfilled expectations had initiated one of many governmental crises in the Philippines.

These days, worldwide, a hundred thousand tons of glucose isomerase and a dozen million tons of fructose syrup are produced annually, and the Yankees are the biggest customers. One kilogram of immobilized enzyme can produce an amazing 20 tons of syrup!

In truth, Coca Cola and Pepsi owe a lot to "El Máximo Líder"!

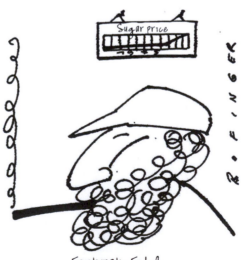

Fortunate Fidel

Chapter 8

Killing Nemo

The movie about the little clownfish Nemo from Pixar Animation Studios is a hilarious and adventure-filled tale, and children can learn a lot from it about life around the world's coral reefs. So taken by the picture were the people of Hong Kong that they bought clownfish for their little ones in droves. Never mind that they are also "enemy number one" of the cute little Nemos: in Asian fish restaurants, you'll find these exquisite reef dwellers in aquariums as a "bycatch". Seafood has to be fresh for the Chinese (a sensible enough philosophy) and besides, the bigger the fish, the easier it is to impress your business partners.

But how do these great creatures wind up in aquariums, alive and without ugly scars from the fishhook? The answer: A poor fellow in Indonesia or in the Philippines dives the coral reefs, armed with a plastic bottle filled with a cyanide solution. He swims to the unwitting fish and forces the cyanhydric acid into their mouths and gills.

One salt of cyanhydric acid, potassium cyanide, is a poisonous gas with a history. The German Nobel Prize winner Otto Warburg discovered in 1926 that cyanide attaches itself to metals, at their oxygen binding sites, for example, to the iron in hemoglobin and respiratory enzymes. The Nazis used cyanhydric acid in the form of Cyclone B (B stands for *blausäure*, German for cyanhydric acid) for the gas chambers in Majdanek and Auschwitz. A tragic irony is that the German-Jewish Nobel Prize winner Fritz Haber, the "father" of the Haber–Bosch process and the devastating "gas war" of WWI, developed the process to be used as insecticide. Many of Haber's relatives died in the concentration camps that used Cyclone B.

Well, being an avid diver, I find this method of fishing quite shocking. Poisoned with cyanide, the fish frantically leave their hiding places in and around the reef in search of fresh, oxygenated water. Giants like Napoleon fish, which are one to two meters in length, are totally powerless and can be dragged by hand to a waiting boat. After this ordeal, they are immediately placed in untainted water, and if they survive, their enzymes will degrade the cyanide. They will quickly be

Who Cloned My Cat? Fun Adventures in Biotechnology by R. Renneberg
Copyright © 2011 by Pan Stanford Publishing Pte Ltd
www.panstanford.com
978-981-4267-65-6

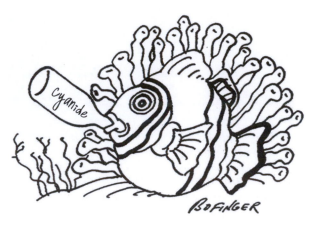

flown to Hong Kong, Singapore and other cities. The cyanide in the fish is not harmful to customers; bitter almonds contain much more cyanhydric acid than such fish.

The result? Because the adult fish are the sole target, and they are removed, there are no juveniles. The cloud of cyanide stays in the reef and poisons small creatures as well, and as the stretches of dead coral expand, the "fishermen" move on to the untouched reefs. It is indeed fortunate that — at least for the moment — there are still some left.

For years, laboratories in the affected countries have been analyzing fish exports in an effort to control the trade. So how do such dealers prove that their fish are cyanide free? "In two minutes, or not at all!" an eyewitness from the Philippines told me. "Go to the person in charge, and in their room you'll see a drawer that happens to have been left open. Throw in a small (or big) donation and — there you go! — you'll get a stamp. Although there is no guarantee that you'll get it." Then he added carefully, "But maybe it was all just a dream I had."

In most cases, the cyanide inside the fish has gone by the time measurements are taken, and the process is so inaccurate that successful detection with the standard method (distillation and a cyanide electrode) would be pure luck.

Our university groups have now developed a highly sensitive enzyme test. But the otherwise very correct Hong Kong authorities were not thrilled when I showed them our cyanide test. "The price of fish will skyrocket, and we all love to eat fish!" was the friendliest comment. Indeed, cyanide fishermen can catch an awful lot more fish in a short period in comparison to those with fishing rods and nets. It is just too easy: poison and grab!

So what does Germany have to do with all this? It is a nation of aquarium lovers. But even aquarium fish are increasingly caught using the cyanide method, mainly for export to the US. And to all those who have an official certificate proclaiming your fish to be "cyanide free," don't be too proud of yourselves. As we've seen, proving the absence of cyanide is an inexact science.

Meanwhile, our work is still ongoing. Together with a fellow scientist from the Tottori University of Japan, we discovered a new enzyme that releases cyanide from the fish's respiratory system, making it possible to detect.

Analytical biotechnology may be the last hope for Nemo and his friends. But time is rapidly running out.

Chapter 9

007 and the Soup Stock

On Her Majesty's secret service in Japan, James Bond (played by the unforgettable Sean Connery) prevents nothing less than another World War in one of the first movies in the franchise. A conflict between the Soviet Union and the US is about to break out over the disappearance of some spaceships. Bond, disguised as a businessman, secretly orders a few tonnes of the chemical substance MSG — spelling out the word *"mono-so-dium-glu-tama-te"* with comic purposefulness. I guess only a few people got the joke back then; basically the same stuff — in the form of "natrium glutamate" — is the ubiquitous ingredient in the powdered soup stock you can buy anywhere around the world!

The flavor enhancer glutamate was identified in 1908 in a seaweed (*Laminaria japonica*) from the Pacific. The salt of L-glutamic acid was found to greatly enhance the taste of soups and sauces. Japanese researcher, Kikunae Ikeda, labeled the taste using the Japanese word "umami" — neither salty nor sweet, neither bitter nor sour. Before then, people had used just these four basic tastes to describe all the sensations detected by the human tongue.

From 1909, the Japanese company Ajinomoto (meaning "the essence of taste") began extracting L-glutamate through fermentation. In Japan, China and Korea, mold fungi and their enzymes (starch-degrading amylases, protein-degrading proteases) have been used for hundreds of years to prepare protein-rich soybeans (protein content: 35 percent) and rice for further processing by alcoholic or lactic fermentation. Soy sauce is made from a mixture of soy and wheat in combination with *Aspergillus oryzae* or *Aspergillus soyae*. In addition to being 18 percent table salt, it contains over one percent glutamate and two percent alcohol.

The demand for glutamate rose dramatically after WWII with the introduction of ready-to-eat meals, gravy powder and premade seasoning. In Japan, they looked for new ways to compensate for the lack of amino acids in the diets of their undernourished population. They turned out to be very successful (see Chap. 71, *Amino Acids, not Made in Japan!* p. 155) and the bio-industry was soon established.

Who Cloned My Cat? Fun Adventures in Biotechnology by R. Renneberg
Copyright © 2011 by Pan Stanford Publishing Pte Ltd
www.panstanford.com
978-981-4267-65-6

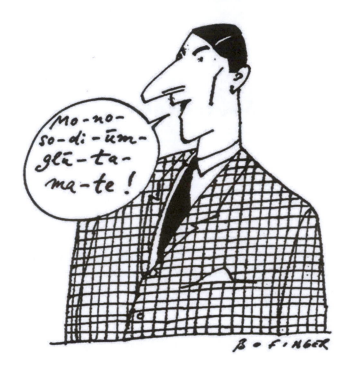

In 1957, the Japanese Shukuo Kinoshita from a rival company, Kyowa Hakko, was testing bacteria and found one that accumulated glutamate when grown on glucose. Named *Corynebacterium glutamicum*, the bacterium allowed the production of glutamate to become much more efficient.

These days, glutamate production exceeds over 1,000,000 tons per year, produced particularly by the Japanese and increasingly by the Chinese bio-industries. The bacteria now produce up to 150 grams of glutamate per liter of bio-culture. Despite prices being slashed to around one US dollar per kilogram, the current market is worth billions.

So take note all those who are allergic to glutamate. My Chinese friends think that only an unskilled cook adds glutamate to their dishes to make them taste better. But around 10 liters of soy sauce is consumed every year in Japan, per person (!) — without any problem.

Scientific opinion varies regarding the "Chinese restaurant syndrome." Some say that it's just psychological. But certainly for some of the "long noses" among my friends in Hong Kong, MSG presents serious problems: prickly skin, heart palpitations and headaches. A Japanese colleague, who is adamant that MSG isn't an issue (provided it comes from Japan), told me: "So what? It's like the feeling you get when you're falling in love."

Chapter 10

Glow, Little Fish, Glow!

After the animated hero Nemo, another fish — this time a real one — caused an uproar in the US. An aquarium fish that glows an attractive bright red color when exposed to ultraviolet light became the first genetically modified pet.

Biotechnologists' love affair with light began about 20 years ago. They succeeded in smuggling a gene from the firefly luciferase (the enzyme used for bioluminescence) into tobacco plants. As the plants were watered, activating the luciferin substrate, the luciferase began to change, and the transgenic plant glowed a greenish yellow.

The experiment was, of course, not designed to allow tobacco to be harvested at night or to create Christmas trees that glow in the dark (see Chap. 42, *Clone Trees*

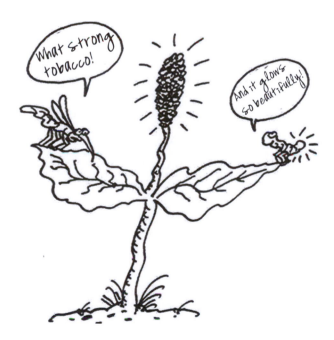

Who Cloned My Cat? Fun Adventures in Biotechnology by R. Renneberg
Copyright © 2011 by Pan Stanford Publishing Pte Ltd
www.panstanford.com
978-981-4267-65-6

That Glow, p. 89). The luciferase gene was used as a marker to determine which genes had been switched on in which parts of the plant. Two scientists from Munich, Eckard Wolf and Alexander Pfeifer, kept 26 luminous green piglets that carry the genes of the Mauve stinger jellyfish. Again, the light emission is used as a genetic marker.

Researchers in Singapore tried to engineer the black-and-white-striped zebrafish (*Danio rerio*) from the Ganges river in India. Their aim is to have the fish glow green (courtesy of the Mauve stinger) or red (from the sea anemone) depending on whether the fish are under stress due to heavy metals in the water or because of the presence of female sexual hormones (estrogens).

The Taiwanese and the Americans have made luminous pets big business: enter the *GloFish*® — sold for around five dollars each. This rapid commercialization caused a good deal of concern among the scientific community. None of the three US oversight boards involved were able to — or wanted to? — prevent distribution, possibly because no-one felt they should be held responsible for the issue.

The US Environmental Protection Agency stayed out of it ("Tropical aquarium fish are not a threat to the environment!") along with the US Food and Drug Administration ("Tropical aquarium fish are not drugs!") and the US Department of Agriculture ("Tropical aquarium fish are not food!"). The "glowfish" was swimming in a regulatory vacuum.

Even if this problem could be resolved, many concerns and questions remain. The fight for approval has been particularly concerned with "size". Take for example the transgenic Pacific salmon (with added growth hormone). They are 11 times bigger than normal, some even 37 times; wild salmon look like midgets by comparison. The other target area is "toughness": economically attractive fish species are supplied with a gene — an anti-freeze protein — to keep them alive in the cold waters of the Arctic.

Besides, who can guarantee that they won't escape from the farm one day? Transgenic cows and pigs can't go back to the wild too easily; the butcher and hungry people see to that. But it's a completely different story with fish!

A disturbing example (not involving gene technology) is the Nile perch (*Lates niloticus*), which was released into Lake Victoria in Africa with the best intentions, but which has displaced nearly all of the local fish species, most significantly the famous Victoria cichlids, and driven them to extinction. The great biologist Charles Darwin never knew about Lake Victoria and its rich diversity of fish. Now, in the blink of an eye, this unique biotope — "Darwin's dream lake," a modern laboratory to study evolution — has been recklessly destroyed by a foreign competitor.

Researchers from Purdue University (West Lafayette, USA) have been experimenting with transgenic fish for a long time. They found that in a Japanese relative of the salmon, called medaka, transgenic males are clearly superior to their wild counterparts: they fertilize eggs at four times the normal rate. As a result, in no more than fifty generations, wild medakas will be wiped out completely.

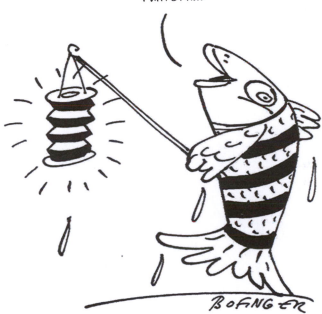

Chapter 11

Aspartame: Nothing but Sweetness

It may be macabre but for the first time in human history the numbers of under- and *over*-nourished people have broken even. So what hope for the world's rotund? Low-calorie sweeteners may be the answer.

In 1965, James Schlatter, a chemist working for the US pharmaceutical firm G. D. Searle, was testing peptides, short chains composed of different amino acids, for the treatment of gastric ulcers. In the lab one day, he accidentally spilled a drop of one of his preparations on his hand. Later, according to one version of the story, as he was trying to pick up some small pieces of paper, he absentmindedly licked his fingertip; it tasted sweet. (Others claim that it happened as he was lighting a cigarette, something that should have been strictly forbidden in the laboratory.) It would turn out that the compound had 200 times the sweetening power of beet or cane sugar.

This new "super sugar," aspartame, is a peptide, a methyl ester from two amino acids, L-asparagine and L-phenylalanine. Both can be produced by bacteria or enzymatically in bioreactors. Although aspartame is broken down by digestive enzymes in the intestines, one gram of aspartame, which equates to an adult's daily intake, only yields four kilocalories — not even one hundredth of the energy humans usually get from sugar. The other good thing about aspartame is that it tastes almost like sugar (aside from the lack of "body"), unlike its rivals saccharin and cyclamate, which have a "metallic" aftertaste.

Saccharin was discovered by a German scientist, Constantin Fahlberg, in 1879. As the "sugar of the poor" it was a triumph, particularly during WWII. Americans Ludwig Audrieth and Michael Sveda discovered cyclamate in 1937 — apparently after Sveda put a cigarette that had been lying on the laboratory bench back in his mouth. Another fortuitous coincidence! Were scientists all smoking in their laboratories back then?

Aspartame, distributed under the name NutraSweet®, hit the market at just the right time. Fitness fever was gripping 1970's America, and with the middle class celebrating crudité parties and jogging to the shops clutching a calorie list,

Who Cloned My Cat? Fun Adventures in Biotechnology **by R. Renneberg**
Copyright © 2011 by Pan Stanford Publishing Pte Ltd
www.panstanford.com
978-981-4267-65-6

aspartame's success was all but guaranteed. These days, 10,000 tons are manufactured worldwide annually.

Soft drinks like Pepsi Cola® use pure aspartame, and in Coca-Cola Light®, it is mixed with other sweeteners. Aspartame has also been sanctioned for use as a food additive. However, patients with the genetic disorder phenylketonuria (0.006 percent of the population) should be cautious since aspartame contains the amino acid phenylalanine, which sufferers must stringently avoid. The Coca-Cola company uses a special label to warn consumers.

So, no calories and no cavities either. Just like the slogan "zero sugar" says? Many experts maintain that this is too good to be true. They argue that by consuming such "light" products, the body expects an inflow of energy, and when that isn't provided, ravenous hunger results. Indeed, it is always with slight trepidation that I watch my (still!) slender Chinese students queuing up for McDonald's at the campus.

Aspartame is, as mentioned above, 200 times sweeter than beet sugar. Cyclamate is 40 times sweeter, acesulfame 200 times, and saccharin some 450 times sweeter. However, all of them have an artificial flavor, and mostly, different sweeteners have to be mixed to try and attain the taste of real sugar.

An even sweeter protein is found in katemfe fruits from a bush plant (*Thaumatococcus danielli*) that grows in West Africa. Called thaumatin (and distributed as Talin®), this sweetener consists of 208 amino acids and is supposedly 2,500 times sweeter than cane sugar. As the recovery of the compounds from this arrowroot plant is very expensive, attempts are being made to produce them using genetically modified microbes.

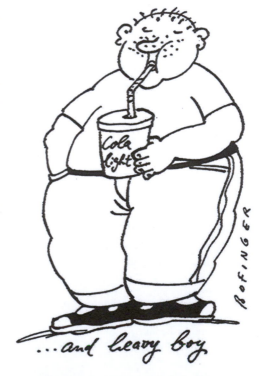

Lots of animals love thaumatin. Its strong smell is the reason why it is found in certain brands of cat food — and why some cats have such a healthy appetite for it. There's little doubt that for some cat food companies, it's the sweet smell of success.

These days there's a new coke available called "Coke Zero" that is marketed as having no sugar whatsoever. It contains both aspartame and acesulfame. Bad times for heavy boy…

…and heavy boy

Chapter 12

"Irasshaimase, Baioteku"

"Irasshaimase, baioteku!" (Welcome, biotechnology!) A delicate Japanese hand passes me a blue carnation. I'm at BIO EXPO JAPAN, one of the most visited exhibitions in Tokyo. I walk a few paces, and I am informed that I just happily accepted a real transgenic plant — like all the other visitors. Apparently, the blue gene from petunias was transplanted into white carnations. Blue roses are the next vision of the Japanese whiskey company Suntory, who of course have advertisements for "Santori orudo uisuki" (Suntory Old Whiskey) at every turn. Some Japanese families are sitting at tables practicing *ikebana* (the Japanese art of flower arrangement) with these transgenic carnations, which supposedly last longer than their standard cousins. At the train station, one will set you back 400 yen (about 3 euros).

Meanwhile, Japanese biotechnologists have embarked on a charm offensive after genetically modified tomatoes and rice got the thumbs down from the majority of consumers. Genetically modified salmon, on the other hand, is awaiting approval to flood the market. Koji Murofushi, a Japanese hammer-throwing Olympian, who won the gold medal in Athens, hasn't been put off though. He consumes a biotechnologically produced amino acid from the food production company Ajinomoto: it's a food supplement — not doping!

Japan is still "No. 1" when it comes to amino acid production, despite stiff competition from China (see Chap. 71, *Amino Acids, not Made in Japan!* p. 155). Murofushi's victory drink, "Amino Vital," which is composed of proteins such as proline, alanine, leucine, isoleucine, valine, glutamate and all the important vitamins, was certainly a great pick-me-up for the tired visitors to the expo hall — me included. You'll find other amino acids in skin creams and shampoos.

Enzymes (*koso* in Japanese) have long been accepted in Japan: Japanese washing machines have always washed with lukewarm water, which is why proteases, amylases and lipases are needed to quickly break down the stains caused by proteins, starch and grease even at low temperatures. Their washing powder is called *koso pawa* (meaning "enzyme power") (see Chap. 45, *Molecular Laundresses*, p. 95, and Chap. 75, *Yams and Cortisone*, p. 165).

Who Cloned My Cat? Fun Adventures in Biotechnology by R. Renneberg
Copyright © 2011 by Pan Stanford Publishing Pte Ltd
www.panstanford.com
978-981-4267-65-6

Other enzymes can dissolve bioplastics in a couple of minutes. In Japan you can find backpacks made of polylactate (PLA) and even biodegradable, but sturdy, rope. Imagine garbage bags and plastic cutlery that break down and disappear after three or four weeks (see Chap. 5, *Computers on the Compost Heap*, p. 9).

Japan is also a leader in biosensor production. The glucose biosensor was simultaneously developed in the mid-1970s in Japan and in the former German Democratic Republic. Back then, East Germany was for a brief time one of the world's best in such technologies. Today, portable glucose biosensors and genetically produced insulin are a must for most diabetic patients.

If it's a handy gimmick you're after, try "biosensor-chopsticks," which warn against too much glutamate. Or how about an "intelligent bio-water closet" for the elderly, which automatically measures the glucose levels in urine? In cases of emergency, the device can even alert the hospital. But if you want to avoid having an ambulance on your doorstep, don't throw leftover beer down your toilet!

In only five minutes, you can monitor your dental health too — one drop of saliva is enough to detect the *Streptococcus mutans* bacteria, which is responsible for tooth decay. Regular brushing with enzyme toothpaste should do the trick!

Kikkoman, famous for its soy sauce, has also jumped on the GM bandwagon and shown that it can shine. One demonstration took place in a darkened room as their champagne was poured into the glasses of a champagne pyramid and began to fluoresce! The spectacle was made possible by the firefly enzyme luciferase in this very unique genetically engineered beverage.

Japanese biotechnologists recognize that "fun" is the name of the game when it comes to selling GM and that they have to do something compelling to gain mass appeal. "The Japanese, they have it easier," complains one German exhibitor.

For the Japanese, getting a positive message across starts with the youngsters. In one of the BIO-Japan rooms, groups of children string colorful pearls together on wires. They learn that on one side the blue A(denin) pearl and the yellow T(hymine) pearl, and on the other side the green C(ytosine) pearl and the red G(uanine) pearl, belong together — and a miniature DNA double helix soon takes shape. Don't be afraid of DNA, kids!

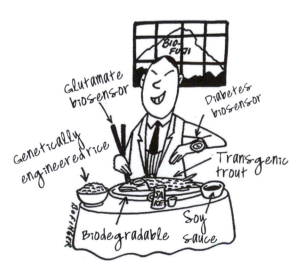

"And when are you going to create a Bio-Fuji?" I ask my Japanese fellow professors jokingly. But it seems some things aren't meant to be made light of. "Fuji-san is the holy mountain and it shall be spared biotechnology. Please just enjoy its beauty!" is the humorless reply.

Chapter 13

Vitamin C and the Fly

In 1933, exciting news came from the basement laboratories of ETH Zurich, Switzerland's premier institute of technology: vitamin C (or L-ascorbic acid) had been successfully synthesized.

Polish-born Tadeusz Reichstein (1897–1996) first chemically degraded glucose in more than ten intermediate stages. The resulting xylose was then converted into vitamin C using hydrogen cyanide. Unfortunately, this method proved far too complex for mass production and only resulted in a small yield. After all, vitamin C is required by the body in larger quantities than any other vitamin.

Reichstein and his young colleague Grüssner decided to try an alternative route. Initially, they wanted to produce sorbose as an intermediate product, but that too proved to be very complicated. Later, they came across the French chemist Gabriel Bertrand's (1867–1962) observation from 1896: the acetic acid-producing bacterium *Acetobacter suboxydans* converts sorbitol into sorbose. Reichstein then did something very unusual for a chemist in his time. Thinking "biotechnologically," he bought some pure cultures of *Acetobacter* from some microbiologists. However, having very limited knowledge of microbiology, he was unable to make use of the bacteria.

Fortunately, Bertrand had also discovered another method to capture the "wild" sorbose bacteria. Fifty years later, Reichstein recalled what the Frenchman wrote: "Take some wine, add a little sugar and vinegar and let it stand in a glass for a day. This mixture will attract swarms of tiny flies called *Drosophila* or fruit flies, which have bacteria in their intestines. As the flies suck up the liquid, they excrete these bacteria, which then start to produce sorbose.

It was late autumn by the time Reichstein planned his experiment, and the fruit flies were nowhere to be seen. However, the weather was still fine and he didn't want to wait until the following summer. So, he gave it a try anyway: "Instead of sugar, I added sorbitol to the wine. I added vinegar as instructed, but I also added some yeast bouillon. I put out five beakers of this mixture on the windowsill in front of my basement laboratory, which just catches a few rays of

Who Cloned My Cat? Fun Adventures in Biotechnology by R. Renneberg
Copyright © 2011 by Pan Stanford Publishing Pte Ltd
www.panstanford.com
978-981-4267-65-6

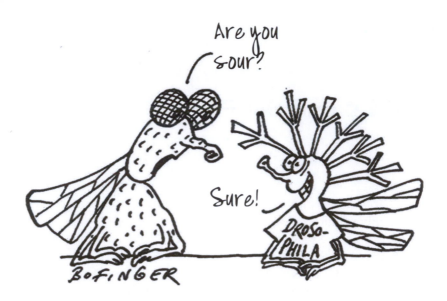

sunshine. That was on a Saturday, and I thought 'Well, if the flies come, that's fine; if they don't, there's nothing to lose.' When I came back on Monday, everything had dried up, but two of the beakers were full of crystals. We studied the crystals and found they were pure sorbose! In one of the beakers, we also found a *Drosophila* specimen that had drowned, and extending from it were rays of sorbose crystals. Those wild bacteria managed to produce more sorbose in two days than the purchased ones could in six weeks!"

He went on: "Converting sorbose into vitamin C was very easy. We could immediately obtain it by the gram and could already predict that it would be possible to produce it by the ton. I think we managed to get 30 to 40 grams of vitamin C out of 100 grams of glucose. Fabulous!" Scientific discovery is a fascinating business — not to mention the sometimes unorthodox methods!

The Roche company in Zürich, which was a fairly small firm back then, took over the license to produce vitamin C from Reichstein — despite mutterings that it was not a pure "chemical" process. To this Reichstein commented sharply: "Like it or not, this bacterium is the only lab assistant capable of achieving a 90 percent sorbose yield from sorbitol. No human can match that! The bacterium does it in two days using nothing but air. All you have to do is feed it some yeast."

Hoffman-La Roche was the world leader in vitamin C production for decades. These days, though, 65 percent is produced by Chinese biotech firms, which churn out vitamin C considerably below the global market price.

Tadeusz Reichstein was awarded the Nobel Prize for Medicine in 1950 — for his work on cortisone, a hormone produced by the cortex of the adrenal gland (see Chap. 75, *Yams and Cortisone*, p. 165).

So, dear readers, when you see some fruit flies circling your fruit basket, don't be too hard on them!

Chapter 14

Magic Bullets Against Cancer

Opera buffs will be familiar with the plot of German Composer Carl Maria von Weber's "Der Freischütz," where the young ranger, Max, tries to get hold of the magic bullets cast in the wolf's glen — magic bullets that cannot fail to find their target.

Magic bullets also fascinated German scientist Paul Ehrlich (1854–1915). Dreaming of using antibodies as the basis for a whole new generation of highly selective drugs, he developed arsphenamine (under the trade name Salvarsan®), a chemotherapeutic drug to cure syphilis. A century has passed since he spoke of his vision of antibodies as magic bullets. Now it finally seems to have come true.

Monoclonal antibodies are very important in modern medicine. Take a viral infection like AIDS for example: antibodies against HIV can be used to identify the virus in the bodily fluids of patients. Such tests have already become routine. Monoclonal antibodies are also used in heart attack and pregnancy tests (see Chap. 15, *Helping Hands for Your Heart*, p. 31 and Chap. 64, *Much Smoke About the Heart*, p. 141). But tests alone don't provide the cure.

It seems, though, that an antibody targeting a certain kind of cancer — non-Hodgkin's lymphoma (NHL) — has been found. NHL is a malignant disease of lymphatic tissue that can affect various parts of the body, such as lymph nodes, the spleen, the thymus gland, the tonsils or bone marrow. Worldwide, around 1.5 million people suffer from NHL and 300,000 die every year. The number of cases increases by three to seven percent annually. In the US, the incidence of NHL is increasing second fastest among cancers — third fastest in the rest of the world. NHL is mostly diagnosed in adults from 45 to 60 years old.

Antibodies to treat NHL can be produced in bioreactors from the fusion of myeloma (cancer) and spleen cells from mice. They are selected specifically so that they only stay at the surface of the cancer cell. Initially, a piggyback toxin (e.g., ricin from the castor oil plant) was used to destroy target cells, but this proved to be no breakthrough as too many healthy cells were damaged in the process.

Who Cloned My Cat? Fun Adventures in Biotechnology **by R. Renneberg**
Copyright © 2011 by Pan Stanford Publishing Pte Ltd
www.panstanford.com
978-981-4267-65-6

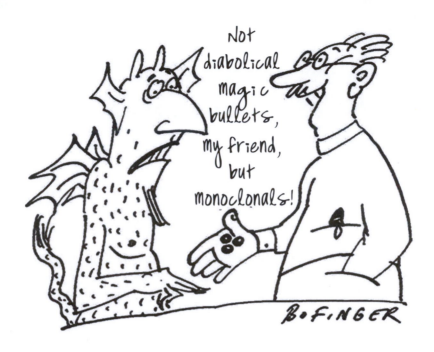

Progress was made once monoclonal antibodies could be genetically modified. The recombinant antibody rituximab ("-mab" stands for monoclonal antibody) interacts exclusively with cells that carry CD20, a protein found at the surface of NHL tumor cells. Rituximab binds to them through various mechanisms that activate the body's own immune system, killing the cell.

Due to its targeted effects, rituximab is well tolerated by patients. It is also one of the first "humanized" recombinant antibodies: proteins of human origin are genetically inserted so that after an injection of rituximab the body does not treat it as foreign and therefore does not elicit an immune response. Rituximab was one of the first hopes, and remains one of the most important treatments, for NHL.

Attempts are being made to reduce the cost of monoclonal antibody production by using milk from transgenic goats or (somewhat more ethically sound) genetically modified plants. Perhaps also bananas — after losing their symbolic power following the reunification of Germany — can regain their luster if researchers can fulfill their dreams of producing monoclonal antibodies from them. Eating the yellow fruit may one day make you immune to cholera or caries-causing bacteria.

I have become a wiser *Ossie* (as we former East Germans have been called): the first thing I did was plant a small banana grove in my garden in Hong Kong. Now I am a self-sufficient producer — no longer beholden to the world's banana distributors!

P.S.: The sales of rituximab climbed to 2 billion US dollars in 2006. So far 300,000 patients have been treated.

Chapter 15

Helping Hands for Your Heart

"Test your blood for the sake of your heart. Results in just 5 minutes!" goes the Dortmund Kuckelke drugstore advertisement. I am currently visiting the world's biggest medical trade fair, MEDICA, in Düsseldorf, Germany, and my biotechnologist's mind cannot say no to the offer.

Ten minutes later, for 15 euros, I'm offered the comforting result: my total cholesterol level is 205 milligrams per deciliter — a little on the high side but these days everyone knows that a high cholesterol level alone does not say much about the risk of arteriosclerosis. Indeed, the levels of various lipids in the blood have to be measured.

No problem: a small device from Taunus micro-medical instruments can quickly read them off a test chip. My triglyceride level, my "good" cholesterol level (high density lipoprotein, or HDL), my "bad" cholesterol level (low density lipoprotein, or LDL) and my very low density lipoprotein level (VLDL) are all within the allowed ranges. The all-important parameter, my total cholesterol/HDL ratio, is exactly 4.0 — right at the limit. Higher levels would indicate a risk of arteriosclerosis.

The friendly pharmacist tries to comfort me. I should have done the test on an empty stomach: the fried egg I had this morning ruined my lipid levels. "Please come again after skipping breakfast!" Hmmm, is it really worth spending another 15 euros when there's basically nothing wrong with me?!

The next generation of rapid tests are on show at MEDICA. Huge automated analyzers for use in hospitals and major laboratories can measure hundreds of substances simultaneously. There is, however, a clear trend towards decentralization and rapid testing on location, so-called point-of-care (POC) testing.

Handy glucose biosensors can now be found in every drugstore. Diabetic patients can measure their glucose levels in seconds without leaving their homes. Leipzig-based SensLab GmbH has a lactic acid sensor that measures the fitness of athletes and the sport inclined. Trained muscle cells aerobically break down glucose better than untrained ones, resulting in less lactic acid production — a sign

Who Cloned My Cat? Fun Adventures in Biotechnology by R. Renneberg
Copyright © 2011 by Pan Stanford Publishing Pte Ltd
www.panstanford.com
978-981-4267-65-6

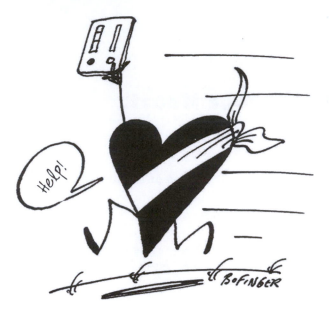

that someone is fit. Anyone can follow their fitness progression with such sensors. We have used the same sensors to measure fitness in racehorses in Hong Kong (in parallel with doping controls) — with great success. Want to bet that someone gets an idea from that?

Other rapid testing indicates the presence of acute myocardial infarction (AMI), otherwise known as a heart attack. Rennesens GmbH from Berlin-Buch have enhanced their "life-saving credit card." Not only is it the world's fastest test for detecting a heart attack early in the life-saving window, but it now also signals older infarctions.

How can we predict a heart attack or stroke before it happens? Warning signals come from inflammation markers. C-reactive protein (CRP) has been recognized in the US as a further risk indicator in addition to blood lipid levels. Several companies offer rapid tests for CRP at the trade fair.

There is another important test to tell a patient with a runny nose and a fever whether they have a viral or a bacterial infection. The test aims to stop the inappropriate use of antibiotics as it is generally known that antibiotics are effective in bacterial infections only. Over-prescribing antibiotics as well as patients deciding to stop taking them as soon as the symptoms disappear have resulted in resistant bacterial strains. New antibiotics or higher doses are then needed — a vicious cycle.

In Hong Kong, when you go to the doctor with a cold, you come away with a whole handful of antibiotic prescriptions. I found it unbelievable. The result: Hong Kong hospitals play host to the world's most dangerously resistant strains of staphylococcus bacteria — the methicillin-resistant *Staphylococcus aureus* (MRSA).

Hopefully, the new tests will cut down the unneccessary usage of antibiotics. That would make our health ministers happy but certainly not the pill-producing pharmaceutical industry.

Chapter 16

Nights on the Highway

In 1985, Dr. Kary Mullis, who was working for the biotech firm Cetus, was on his way home for the weekend, zipping along the California highway. Cetus, Latin for "whale," was the world's first modern biotech company. During those three long hours on that moon-lit highway, he thought about how one could produce millions or even billions of copies of a specific DNA fragment.

Mullis watched the lights of the cars going in different directions, meeting, passing each other and heading off at the various junctions. This symphony of interweaving lights sparked an idea. He stopped his car, woke up his sleeping girlfriend, and began to draw lines showing how DNA duplicates itself in the test tube — the product of each cycle providing material for the next. Just 20 cycles would be enough to generate 1,000,000 identical DNA molecules! "Darling, I may get the Nobel Prize!", he explained to his surprised girlfriend.

Back at the Cetus laboratory on Monday, Mullis began working feverishly on his new idea, and it worked! However, his colleagues were not terribly impressed.

It was such a simple idea; surely somebody somewhere must have tried it out before. Soon afterwards, Nobel Prize winner and Cetus consultant Joshua Lederberg took a careful look at the poster Mullis was presenting at a conference, and asked more or less in passing, "Does it work?" Mullis nodded and finally got the reaction he had hoped for. The iconic giant of molecular genetics tore at his thinning hair and exclaimed, "Oh my god, why didn't I think of that?"

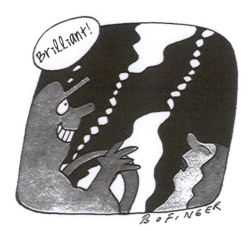

I've heard the same reactions from my colleagues in the former East

Who Cloned My Cat? Fun Adventures in Biotechnology by R. Renneberg
Copyright © 2011 by Pan Stanford Publishing Pte Ltd
www.panstanford.com
978-981-4267-65-6

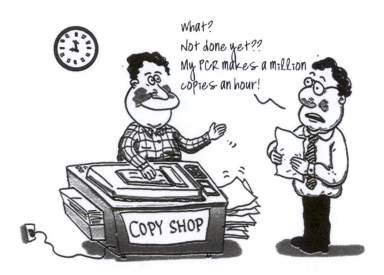

Germany. Tom Rapoport, a friend and colleague from Berlin-Buch, now professor (not at Berlin but at Harvard!), once stormed into a seminar, during East German times, shouting: "The Americans have started a revolution — in the test tube!" Tom himself is a potential Nobelist.

The technique is called the polymerase chain reaction (PCR), and it imitates cell division: as the genetic information provided to each of the daughter cells must be identical, the entire set must be copied from the mother cell. The two strands of the double helix are separated, and both single-stranded DNA molecules serve as templates for the formation of new single strands. An enzyme called DNA polymerase helps synthesize the complementary strands within the cell.

In order to obtain single-stranded DNA from the test tube, it has to be heated to 94°C (201°F) and cooled down again for synthesizing. Boiling hot springs yield microorganisms that also rely on a polymerase for their replication. The polymerase isolated from *Thermus aquaticus* has been genetically modified and produced in large quantities. It works most effectively at 72°C (162°F) and can survive undamaged at 94°C (201°F). Hence, it remains active in the test tube for the whole cycle.

With a cycle lasting just three minutes, in an hour, one million copies can be made from one single DNA! PCR is a DNA-copying mechanism *par excellence*.

PCR is invaluable not only in research but also in diagnostics. Bacteria and viruses can be identified directly: no artificial replication process is required. PCR is increasingly used in the diagnostics of hereditary diseases and cancer. In the fight against crime, a small amount of DNA is multiplied with the help of PCR and later identified through DNA fingerprinting (see Chap. 78, *Genetic Fingerprints*, p. 173).

Kary Mullis earned the Nobel Prize in 1993, only eight years after his epochal discovery.

Chapter 17

Doping? No, caterpillar fungus!

In September 1993, in Beijing a scandal arose during the Chinese National Championships. The favorite, Junxia Wang, ran the 10,000 meters in a world record time of 29:31.78, breaking the sub-30-minute barrier and the earlier record by some 42 seconds. Not long after, the world record for the 1,500 meters was broken by Yunxia Qu, and the 3,000 meters first by Linli Zhang and then again by Junxia Wang (8:06.11). These times remain the current world records.

So many new world records set at the same place in such a short time? Skeptics across the whole world agreed: urine testing would be needed to show the use of doping by female Chinese runners. But the tests were negative. Their coach Zunren Ma pointed to the extreme training at high altitude in Tibet, the great team spirit, Chinese turtle soup (which supposedly regulates menstruation) and a tiny fungus, *Cordyceps sinensis*. Ma used to be a farmer.

My boss at the university, Professor Naiteng Yu, was surprised that I had never heard of the fungus before: "The fungus is called winter-worm summer-plant by the Chinese because we believe that it is an animal in winter and a plant in summer. The fungus has been used for over a thousand years in traditional Chinese medicine. It stimulates the Yang (the concept of heaven from ancient Chinese philosophy) and therefore nourishes the lungs and kidneys. It is taken by people suffering from liver problems, cancer, angina pectoris, heart rhythm problems, sexual problems, hepatitis and tuberculosis."

The magic fungus grows in alpine grasslands in the southwest of China, in Yunnan prefecture, in middle and northern China, and in Tibet at very high altitudes up to 5,000 meters. The fruiting bodies emerge like a finger or a pencil, four to ten centimeters from the soil surface. The fungus leads an extraordinary way of life — by killing caterpillars living underground, feeding off the nutrients and then later sprouting from the surface. It is thought that the caterpillars ingest the fungal spores quite by accident. Cordyceps is closely related to the German *Claviceps purpurea*, a grain fungus that can cause LSD-type effects.

Who Cloned My Cat? Fun Adventures in Biotechnology by R. Renneberg
Copyright © 2011 by Pan Stanford Publishing Pte Ltd
www.panstanford.com
978-981-4267-65-6

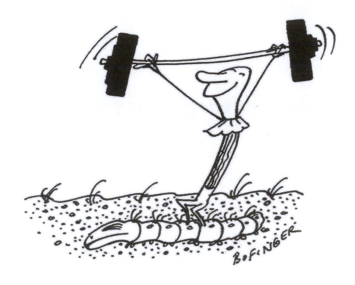

These days, the Chinese caterpillar fungus is hard to find in nature. Professional cordyceps collectors spend their time scouring the country for it; the price per kilogram has risen from 3000 to 5000 US dollars — more expensive than truffles.

The worldwide demand has encouraged cultivation. One biotech company in Hawaii has managed to grow cordyceps successfully by utilizing a cold-storage warehouse to simulate its natural environment in Tibet. Further research has revealed that the underground mycelia (the vegetative part of the fungus) contain an even more effective substance, the extract of which is now sold in capsule form.

Researchers have explained the increased performance in sport as arising from the positive effects of the caterpillar fungus on the respiratory organs and the heart. Aside from vitamins and minerals, it also contains high-quality amino acids like polysaccharides — hence the reason why the tests for performance-enhancing drugs turned out negative.

Studies undertaken by the Medical Faculty in Beijing University have also proven with certainty popular claims in traditional Chinese medicine that caterpillar fungus works as an aphrodisiac (for both men and women) and boosts sexual stamina.

It's still not known how it works. But the fungus certainly has some animal fans: Himalayan yaks are very partial to the fungus and are filled with "natural vigor and vitality" during cordyceps harvesting time. Just as the sexual hormones in truffles excite their swine cousins, caterpillar fungus has given these hardy bovines a true *yakphrodisiac*!

Chapter 18

Running Out of Phosphate

Phosphorous is important: both animals and plants need it as a building block of DNA and — in the form of adenosine triphosphate (ATP) — as "fuel" for the cell. But the widespread use of phosphate in fertilizers and animal feed remains a major environmental concern. Phosphate is one substance that has undergone big changes both in terms of its use and acceptance in the past 100 years. Environmental issues, economic growth and technological advances have defined our view of phosphorus and its salt, phosphate.

Excessive amounts of phosphates and nitrates from agricultural run-off have led to massive water eutrophication — an over-accumulation of nutrients that often results in enormous algae growth. As the algae dies, they are decomposed by bacteria, and this consumes oxygen in the water, which in turn starves fish of oxygen. Anerobic bacteria step in, producing toxic ammonia and hydrogen sulphide, which kills the remaining living creatures. The result is a foul, reeking cesspool.

Algae that differ in color but are equally toxic make up the Red Tides in the southern seas, e.g., in Hong Kong, but they also appeared in Germany's Firth of Kiel years ago. The red-brown color of the water comes from a microscopic organism of the dinoflagellate family (dual-flagellated carapaced algae) that thrives on a combination of warm water and nutrients and produces toxins.

The market is doing what appellants cannot do: the dynamic growth of China and India is leading to uncontrolled surges and fluctuations in raw material prices. In China, animal feeds containing inorganic phosphate have risen 70 percent.

In response, phosphorus is slowly beginning to be "managed," and in the lead role is an enzyme — what else?! — called phytase.

Monogastric animals like chickens, pigs and of course humans discard most of the phosphates they ingest because their stomachs are unable to hydrolyze phytate (phytic acid), the stored form of phosphate in plant seeds. Microorganisms that produce phytase activity, by contrast, inhabit the multi-chambered stomachs of ruminants. The phytase enzyme breaks down the phosphate groups from

Who Cloned My Cat? Fun Adventures in Biotechnology by R. Renneberg
Copyright © 2011 by Pan Stanford Publishing Pte Ltd
www.panstanford.com
978-981-4267-65-6

phytate and makes them bioavailable through hydrolytic cleavage. Phytase is produced by various microbes, including fungi, and excreted extracellularly.

Biotechnologists and animal nutritionists hit on the idea of adding phytase to pig and chicken feed, which resulted in a 25–30 percent reduction in phosphate excretion. The animals' stomachs can digest the phosphate in their feed more easily, and thus less phytase is needed in the feed.

In countries with intensive animal farming like the Netherlands and Denmark, the use of phytase has lowered environmental phosphorous pollution by thousands of tons per year while saving on animal feed as well. Governments there actively encourage its use, as some states in the US are also beginning to do.

Novozymes, a Danish firm, is the world's biggest producer of phytase. They manufacture a phytase preparation from the fungus *Peniophora lycii*. The company has exported in huge quantities to China, but the Chinese are about to take over production themselves. China has wisely cut back on phosphate mining and reduced their domestic use of phosphate in animal feed.

"Green" biotechnology is still making progress: phytase genes can now be genetically inserted into corn, rice and soybeans. Still, as long as green biotech (unlike the medical-oriented variety) continues to struggle for approval in Europe and the US, phytase as an animal feed supplement remains the more successful candidate in the short term.

My Chinese alter ego chastizes me: "You Germans with your paltry population of 80 million! We can't afford such luxury for our 1.3 billion people. They need feeding now! We have to think about the future, too."

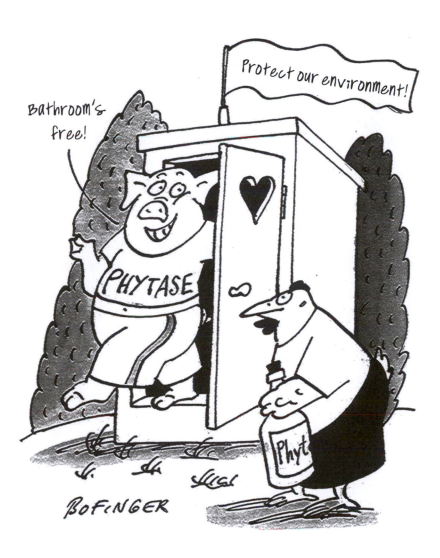

Chapter 19

Snowmax for the Alps?

Most plants cannot survive frost or freezing temperatures. Why is that so? The answer is that the ice crystals forming on the leaves and other parts of the plant destroy the living tissue. Bacteria play the key role in this. These organisms, only a thousandth of a millimeter in size, serve as crystallization nuclei for the ice crystals. Tap water freezes at 0°C (32°F) but purified distilled water can be cooled to −15°C and still remain fluid — as long as it does not contain any impurities to form nuclei for crystallization.

One crystal-forming type of bacteria in particular is widespread in nature: *Pseudomonas syringae*. Biotechnologists Steven Lindow and Nikolas Panopoulos from the US have examined normal plants infected with *Pseudomonas syringae* in a climatic chamber at temperatures below the freezing point. At −2°C (28.4°F), the first frost damage started, but plants where the bacteria had been killed were able to tolerate −8°C (17.6°F) and even −10°C (14°F) without damage. The cause: a special protein on the surface of the tiny organisms that stimulated the formation of ice crystals.

If a section could be cut from a DNA strand of the frost bacteria, containing the command for formation of the frost protein, this would also destroy the capacity for forming ice crystals. Genetically engineered "anti-frost bacteria" achieve just that — protecting their hosts from frost damage. Spraying plants with an inexpensively produced anti-frost bacteria liquid is sufficient as the genetically modified microbes displace the natural ones.

This opens up some attractive approaches. For example, a number of cultivated plants that until now have only

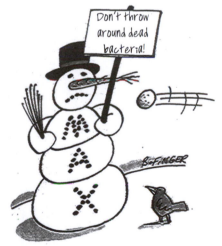

Who Cloned My Cat? Fun Adventures in Biotechnology by R. Renneberg
Copyright © 2011 by Pan Stanford Publishing Pte Ltd
www.panstanford.com
978-981-4267-65-6

thrived in warmer regions can also be grown further north. But how would the newly created microbes behave in the environment? Who could guarantee that weeds and plant pests would not also benefit from the frost protection bacteria? Would the biological balance be disturbed? Once microbes have been released into the environment, they cannot be recalled. After years of debate, it was decided *not* to approve open-air trials with such genetically modified microbes.

So what of the dream? A clever biotechnologist came up with an idea: mass-produce the natural frost bacteria in bioreactors, kill them, and then sell them under the name Snowmax® for the production of artificial snow! With these special dead bacteria added to the water in snow guns, snow production increases by 45 percent. Snowmax® also saves on the energy required for refrigeration. It turns out that no authorities forbade the release of non-manipulated stone-dead microbes.

In the meantime, the "made with Snowmax®" artificial snow business is booming worldwide. Indeed, these dead frost bacteria rescued the 1988 Winter Olympics in Calgary (Canada) during an unexpected warm spell.

As I was browsing through pictures of German winterscapes, I came up with a great business idea: Snowmax® could be used to cover the whole of Hong Kong with snow. On second thought, at 30°C it would all end up as slush in no time. Maybe we should just enjoy the beaches instead!

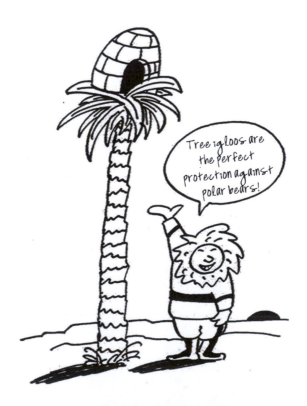

Chapter 20

Praise for the Papaya

When the Spanish conquered Mexico, they noticed that the indigenous people would wrap leaves of the papaya tree (*Carica papaya*) around meat they wanted to cook or fry. Alternatively, they would rub their meat with a slice of unripe papaya fruit or add the latex from this evergreen tree. The natives swore by the magical power of the papaya.

It turns out that none of this was unreasonable as we have now discovered that papayas contain high concentrations of the proteases papain and chymopapain in their latex or fruit flesh. They degrade connective tissue in the meat, making it nice and tender.

Hundreds of tons of papain are used in the US every year for tenderizing meat. Other proteases — ficin from fig trees and bromelain from pineapple plants — are also suitable for the purpose. In tropical countries, papain is used not only to tenderize meat but also as a digestive aid.

Tenderizing powders containing proteases are sold in many countries. They can be rubbed into meat and then left to stand at room temperature for several hours. (Papain remains stable and active even at 80°C.) During this time, plant proteases degrade connective tissue proteins, such as collagen and elastin, speeding up natural maturing processes.

Still, one should remain skeptical about sensationalist advertisements for tenderizers that promise to turn chewy beef into delicious tender veal in minutes. Tenderizers only speed up meat's natural maturing process. Everyone knows that you have to let your meat hang for a while to improve the flavor. The animal's own proteases (cathepsins) are at work in this maturation process.

Strong demand has already led to the first biotechnology-derived papayas being planted in Hawaii. The indigenous people from this archipelago in the Pacific have known about the effects of papaya latex for hundreds of years. Hawaii even has its own "enzyme fairytale," which tells of a hapless hero who one day tries to use the "magical power" of the papaya tree to turn himself into a strong and handsome man in order to win the heart of a beautiful princess.

Who Cloned My Cat? Fun Adventures in Biotechnology by R. Renneberg
Copyright © 2011 by Pan Stanford Publishing Pte Ltd
www.panstanford.com
978-981-4267-65-6

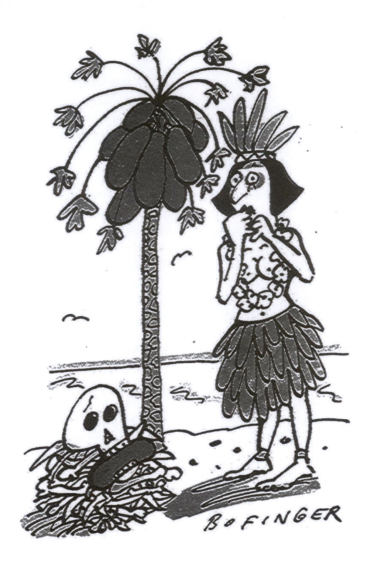

In the shade of a papaya tree, our pitiful hero mixes rice with a huge number of papaya leaves and fruits, and stuffs himself with it — the more the better — until late into the night.

But when his friends come to look for him at his dining spot the next morning, all that's left is a pile of bones...

Most astonishingly of all, according to my trusty encyclopedia, this two-meter killer tree belongs to, of all things, the violet plant family!

I have a papaya tree in my miniature garden in Hong Kong that I planted from a seed, and I have always enjoyed the lovely fragrance from its tiny blossoms. But since hearing about that Hawaiian fairytale, I can't help but eye my fast-growing tree just a little warily.

Chapter 21

Biochemical Bird Market

One of the things I look forward to on the weekend is a visit to Hong Kong's bird market, which seems to reflect life in Hong Kong in microcosm: ten thousand birds packed in small cages, loudly and cheerfully eating and drinking.

The market also serves as a nice analogy for biotechnology — as here the basic principles of "immobilization" are demonstrated quite clearly. Immobilizing means to fix and to make unmovable. Two of the most important ways of fixing enzymes and microbes for use in industry are the embedding method and employing covalent bonds. It's all about somehow immobilizing the biomaterial without blocking its activities. The idea is that enzymes (as well as microbes) continuously turn their substrates into products without ending up in the products themselves. Moreover, the microbial "workers" have to be on duty for as long as possible.

Chinese nightingales are models of immobilized enzymes. They are locked inside beautiful but narrow wooden cages. They can (well, just about) move inside the cage. And they sing beautifully — their "activities" are in full swing! They are provided with the necessary substrate (food, oxygen and water) and they dispose of their "products" in dribs and drabs without escaping from the cage. They are truly "immobilized."

The birds cannot get out of the cage but Mao-jai, the kitten, cannot get in either. In the same way, enzymes must also be protected from other enzymes (e.g., proteases in detergents, see Chap. 45, *Molecular Laundresses*, p. 95 and Chap. 74, *Genetic Engineering in Your Washer*, p. 163) or greedy microbes.

Biosensors use precisely this method. Take for instance glucose biosensors for diabetic patients. Here, the glucose oxidase enzyme is immobilized in a polymer "cage." Glucose in blood and oxygen can enter the cage and the product, hydrogen peroxide, can be diffused out of the cage to an electrode in order to display the glucose content.

We have been developing microbial sensors with Professor Gotthard Kunze from the Institute of Plant Genetics and Crop Plant Research in Gatersleben

Who Cloned My Cat? Fun Adventures in Biotechnology by R. Renneberg
Copyright © 2011 by Pan Stanford Publishing Pte Ltd
www.panstanford.com
978-981-4267-65-6

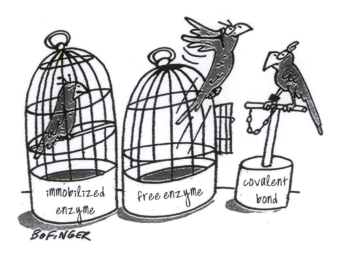

immobilized enzyme

free enzyme

covalent bond

BOFINGER

(Sachsen-Anhalt, Germany). In our sensors, immobilized yeast in polymer cages can measure organic pollution in wastewater. The yeast is "locked up in cages" for months, yet remains active. With this new technology it only takes five minutes to take measurements — compared with five days using traditional methods.

History informs us about how canaries were once used in the West as living biosensors in the coal mining industry to warn miners of flammable gases and poisonous carbon monoxide. A bird passing out was a sign of danger.

Other enzymes have been immobilized for fructose syrup production (see Chap. 7, *How Fidel Saved US Biotech*, p. 13). The glucose isomerase enzyme in its polymer cage is used industrially to convert glucose into fructose with twice the sweetness. Another immobilized enzyme, penicillin acylase, has been used to synthesize a new derivative penicillin that bacteria are (for now) not resistant to.

Alongside Hong Kong's caged birds are the cockatoos and parrots. Prevented from flying away from their perches, they are also immobilized, but with a chain (covalency). This is just how antibodies are immobilized in biotechnology. They can be found in cellulose strips and can bind with, for example, pregnancy hormones, myocardial infarction proteins or drugs — like a sleuthhound on a leash (see Chap. 51, *Academic Dog-Catching*, p. 111).

What else could you immobilize? The aspiring brewer can get lots of ideas from Japan, where immobilized yeast is used to produce alcohol at home. One Japanese cartoon I've seen showed how kitchen waste is converted into alcohol in home bioreactors. It is used as an energy source for cooking (ostensibly for the woman of the house), as a biofuel for the family car (see Chap. 69, *Tanking US with Corn*, p. 151), and also to relax the husband after a long day at the office.

Chapter 22

One Pill for (Almost) Everything?

What is today's most frequently taken medicine? Its use dates back to ancient times: it was even described by Hippocrates. In 1828, a Munich professor called Johann Buchner isolated it from willow bark (*Salix*) as a yellow, crystalline mass, and named it salicin. By 1889 Felix Hoffmann had patented acetylsalicylic acid (ASA), the active component of willow extract, and offered the concept to the Bayer company.

Bayer subsequently created a catchy name for it: "A" from acetyl chloride, combined with "spir" from *Spiraea ulmaria* (or meadowsweet, which also contains salicylic acid) and added the suffix "in" — aspirin. First sold in tablets in 1915, it has been circling the globe at unparalleled speed ever since. It wasn't long before aspirin was being widely used without prescription for all manner of ailments.

So how does aspirin work biochemically? It blocks the production of the body's prostaglandins, the hormones that transfer "messages" locally. Unlike other hormones, prostaglandins only affect surrounding cells. For example, they control the contraction of muscle cells, blood vessels and clumping of blood platelets. Effectively, prostaglandins pass on and strengthen local pain signals.

All prostaglandins come from the conversion of a precursor, arachidonic acid. If this enzyme is inhibited, pain signals do not arise as reactions to inflammation and blood clotting are also delayed. Aspirin does exactly that: it blocks the cyclooxygenase (COX) enzyme.

There are two variations of the enzyme: COX-1, which exists in almost all cells, and COX-2, which can only be found in special cells and which signals inflammation and amplifies pain. Aspirin blocks both forms of cyclooxygenase. This explains the adverse reactions experienced through uncontrolled long-term use: gastric and intestinal bleeding, kidney damage and gastric ulcers. A modern painkiller like Vioxx®, by contrast, only blocks COX-2 and leaves COX-1 alone (see Chap. 41, *Mussel Extract Takes On Vioxx®*, p. 87).

Yet aspirin and other "non-steroidal anti-inflammatories" do more than reduce pain. Research has shown that inflammation blockers are capable of reducing the growth of cancer cells. In animal tests they have slowed down the growth

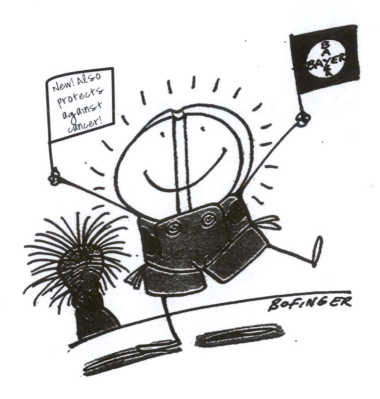

of tumors. Medical observations that began in 1976, carried out by more than 120,000 nurses in the US, have shown that the longer aspirin is regularly taken, the rarer it is that colon cancer develops. However, the detailed protective effects are not yet fully understood.

Moreover, it has been reported in the *Journal of the American Medical Association* (*JAMA*) that women who use aspirin to prevent heart disease registered a positive side effect: aspirin reduced the risk of developing the most widespread type of breast cancer. I personally take a small amount of aspirin every day to make my blood "thinner" and to prevent a heart attack.

A clear conclusion has emerged: aspirin is not a life insurance and it does not help to fight disease; it only reduces the risks — but still! As a miracle cure for heart infarction, it can only prevent the first infarction and cannot eliminate it entirely. Also, its effect on women, as research published in *New England Journal of Medicine* has shown, can be demonstrated only in those over 65 years old.

From a purely economic point of view, aspirin is probably the most cost-effective precaution against disease we have. It can also be locally produced in poorer developing countries — which no doubt irks the pharmaceutical giants.

The World Health Organization mentions acetylsalicylic acid three times in its list of essential medicines. It also points out that aspirin is not a harmless home remedy but a highly effective medicine that should not be taken recklessly.

Speaking of which… I'm starting to get a headache. Where are my magic pills?

Chapter 23

Sterilized to Perfection

Napoleon Bonaparte knew that soldiers could not march well on an empty stomach (and without red wine to disinfect the water!). And so it was that in 1795 he would offer a prize to whoever could find a practical method for preserving food long term. The French chef Nicholas Appert finally came up with a solution after working on the problem for 14 years, and in 1809 he received a prize of 12,000 gold francs — a fortune worth about 250,000 euros or 350,000 US dollars today. The method might appear trivial today: heating food in bottles and jars, sealed with corks. The preserved food would keep for months.

The working principle of vacuum sealing — negative pressure is exerted during cooling, sucking the lid firmly closed — goes back to experiments by Otto von Guericke (1602–1686) and Denis Papin (1647–1712). Guericke's famous 1654 experiment with his so-called Magdeburg hemispheres at the Reichstag in Regensburg demonstrated the enormous power of air pressure: the vacuum contained in the sphere created by pumping out the air was so good that it could not be pulled apart by 16 horses.

Another expert in this field was the German chemist Rudolf Rempel (1850–1893). His invention, which was patented in 1892, was later described by his wife in a letter: "For the first experiments he used the glass jars for powder from the chemistry laboratory whose rims were ground smooth. He equipped the jars with rubber rings and metal lids and cooked the food inside using a water bath with a heavy object (stone or weight) on top of the lid."

Rempel's first successful tests with sterilizing milk widened the experiments, with the help of his wife, to trying to preserve various kinds of produce from their garden. "I ground the glass jars with abrasive powder in the sink, which was a lot of work, and we tried out various methods to sterilize fruits and vegetables. Most of the containers did not close well, but those that did held up nicely." Such experiences can easily be comprehended even today. Ultimately, an apparatus was devised that used a spring to press metal lids onto glass containers.

Who Cloned My Cat? Fun Adventures in Biotechnology **by R. Renneberg**
Copyright © 2011 by Pan Stanford Publishing Pte Ltd
www.panstanford.com
978-981-4267-65-6

You might be wondering what this has to do with biotechnology. Well, the lack of oxygen in the containers prevents the growth of oxygen-requiring (aerobic) microbes like decomposing bacteria and mildew. Such "spoilers" are eliminated to the greatest extent through heating, which drastically lowers their numbers.

One of Rempel's first customers was Johann Weck. He showed great interest in the method; one of his orders included a whole wagon full of jars. Weck acquired the patent from Rempel and in 1895 moved to Öflingen in Germany at the border with Switzerland. With his active business partner Georg van Eyck, they established the company J. Weck & Co on January 1, 1900.

Weck left the company only two years later (due to illness) leaving the production license behind. Van Eyck successfully introduced and sold WECK® jars and canning devices throughout the country. He had an ingenius business model: employ home economics teachers to give lectures in culinary schools, churches and hospitals about practical guidance on how to use the new jars and canning equipment.

The components were constantly improved: the preserve jars and canning devices, the rubber rings, the thermometers and the ancillary equipment — everything under the name WECK® with its strawberry logo. WECK® became Germany's first brand and even spawned the German verb for preserving: *ein*-weck-*en*.

The tradition of "einwecken" is typically German. The Americans, for example, would probably not bother to take the time. The Chinese on the other hand — diligent and business-minded as they are — would probably have earned van Eyck an even bigger profit.

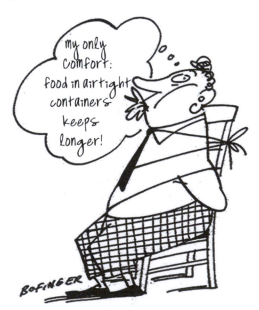

Chapter 24

A Tale About a Cold

During the cherry blossom season, Japan is as beautiful as if in a dream. A long time ago, I was working in Japan as a Post-Doctoral fellow in the old capital, Kyoto. Each year television reports excitedly track the blooming *sakura* (the Japanese word for the cherry blossoms that are so central to Japanese culture) beginning in the south.

Then, all of a sudden, throats begin to itch… and before long a full-blown sore throat develops! But the chemists in Japan have a new remedy at the ready — one is called *Li-so-zi-mu*. This medicine, in the form of lozenges, instantly helps with its *koso pawa* ("enzyme power"; see Chap. 45, *Molecular Laundresses*, p. 95 and Chap. 74, *Genetic Engineering in Your Washer*, p. 163) to fight sore throats.

A cold didn't stop Alexander Fleming (1881–1955) from coming to work in his London laboratory in 1922. One night, he was about to throw away some old Petri dishes, which had been standing around for days, when he realized that one of them looked different. He showed it to his assistant, V. D. Allison, and commented with typical British understatement: "Quite interesting!"

Large yellow bacteria colonies were covering the jelly-like mass, but one spot was free of organisms. A quiz question: What had Fleming discovered? Penicillin? Wrong! That came later. No, indeed, following his researcher's instincts, a few days earlier Fleming had added some mucus from his nose to the center of the bacterial culture, and it was this that had led to the bacteria-free area. Something in the mucus seemed to have killed (or *lysed*) the bacteria.

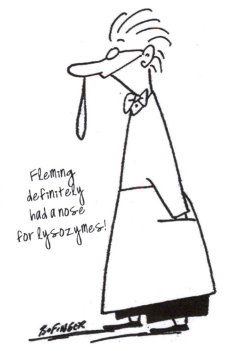

Fleming definitely had a nose for lysozymes!

BoFINGER

Who Cloned My Cat? Fun Adventures in Biotechnology by R. Renneberg
Copyright © 2011 by Pan Stanford Publishing Pte Ltd
www.panstanford.com
978-981-4267-65-6

It could only have been an enzyme that lysed the microbes, so he called it a lysozyme. Fleming later discovered that all bodily fluids contain lysozymes — one example being tears. It wasn't long before he had colleagues and students alike working in the laboratory with red eyes — having aggravated their tear glands with lemons and onions! Even visitors were expected to contribute by providing tears for Fleming's experiments.

Egg white is also rich in lysozymes, which shield chicks from microbial invasion.

The substrate of the lysozyme is a molecule consisting of sugar rings. This mucopolysaccharide serves as a building component of cell walls. When the lysozyme cleaves to its substrate, the cell becomes permeable, takes up liquid and finally bursts from the high osmotic pressure inside.

To Fleming's disappointment, it turned out that the mighty lysozyme was only effective at killing harmless microbes, but it had no effect whatsoever on pathogens. It took a further seven years before Fleming discovered a very effective antibiotic — penicillin — in what seems to be another fortuitous experiment.

"Chance favors the prepared mind." This is how the master of biotechnology, Louis Pasteur, described such a creative process — something that he himself experienced a number of times.

The lysozyme, it turns out, was destined to assume a very special place in the history of modern biology, as it was the first enzyme to have its spatial structure studied and its properties explored in atomic-level detail. With a three-dimensional model, it was possible to show for the first time how a substrate (key) exactly fit in an enzyme (lock).

Today, we know, however, that lysozyme and other enzymes are work via the "induced fit" model: both substrate and enzyme are flexible in shape, like fingers and gloves.

Well, it's about time I had another lysozyme "candy" for my throat… and I'm thinking to myself: those Japanese are actually busy taking stuff invented by us "long noses"!

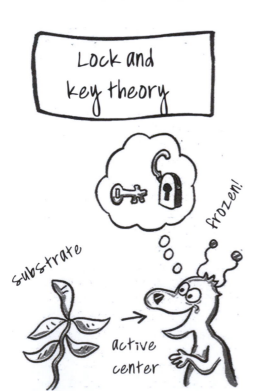

Chapter 25

Biotech at the Barber's?

If there's one place that information flows freely — substantiated or otherwise — it's hair salons. It was where my Hong Kong hairdresser, Ringo, told me about the astonishing things happening in the "motherland," China: "Don't tell anyone — but they eat hair over there! Well, maybe not the hair itself… this is what I heard from a customer."

This was no idle gossip. The truth is that ten thousand tons of hair are swept up by professional collectors every year from China's hair salons and delivered to manufacturers who extract cysteine using activated charcoal and concentrated hydrochloric acid. A sulfur-containing amino acid, cysteine is unique because of its chemically highly reactive sulfhydryl group. By building disulfide bridges, it contributes to the stability of proteins, enabling the formation of strong fibrous strands such as hair, wool and feathers, as well as horns, hooves and nails.

Cysteine is used, for example, as a baking ingredient to facilitate the kneading of dough, or in cough medicines. The cosmetic industry is taking its share, too. Japanese and Hong Kong hairdressers use it in preparations for perms rather than the pungent thioglycolic acid mostly used in Europe. Cysteine is even used to produce artificial meat flavorings. When cysteine binds to a sugar such as ribose, aromatic compounds develop during the heating process — which taste like meat. This imitation of natural processes occurs, for example, when meat is fried. The cysteine present in meat reacts with the sugar to form the characteristic aromatic compounds.

Until very recently, cysteine was one of the few amino acids that could only be extracted from animal and human sources. And extracting cysteine has become big business in Asia: one ton of hair yields 100 kilograms of cysteine. Every year 4,000 tons of cysteine are used globally and the demand is rising at an annual rate of four percent. An alternative production method would be very welcome indeed.

Researchers at the German company Wacker Fine Chemicals have succeeded in programming that biotechnology workhorse, *E. coli* (see also Chap. 27, *Even*

Who Cloned My Cat? Fun Adventures in Biotechnology by R. Renneberg
Copyright © 2011 by Pan Stanford Publishing Pte Ltd
www.panstanford.com
978-981-4267-65-6

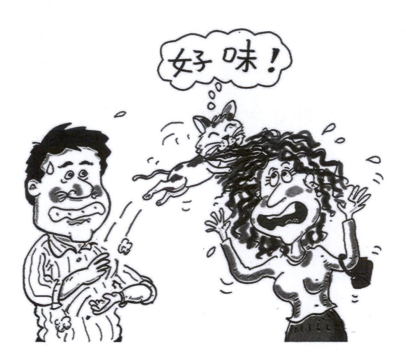

Bacteria Grow Old, p. 57), through targeted mutagenesis and selection so that it produces more cysteine than it needs. This excess cysteine is then put into fermentation vessels for production.

There are several advantages to this biotechnological approach. It is highly efficient (90 percent compared to 60 percent) and the extraction process also uses far less hydrochloric acid (one kilogram of acid per kilogram of extracted cysteine). The end product is 98.5% pure cysteine, which meets all the necessary food and pharmaceutical quality standards. By 2004, more than 500 tons of cysteine had been produced by this method, with an annual growth rate of over 10 percent.

This won't be putting Asian hair collectors out of work anytime soon. There will be a shift in market share, but several thousand tons of cysteine will still be extracted in the conventional way every year.

Customers who care more about price than the product's origin will continue to buy it, for example, to enhance their favorite cat or dog food. Rumors are spreading among cat and dog owners that their beloved pets crave only certain brands.... So don't be surprised if Mao-jai jumps on your fresh perm meowing "Hou mei" (delicious!) after your next visit to the hairdresser's!

Chapter 26

Just as Long as It Catches Mice!

"The color of the cat matters not, as long as it catches mice." With these words Deng Xiaoping once initiated reforms in China. Many cat lovers would beg to differ: they would rather have a perfect copy of their little Monty or Mao-jai after they pass away.

Take Little Nicky, a cute cloned cat, produced by the US company Genetics Savings and Clone and sold for some 50,000 US dollars. It was the first commercially cloned cat but not the first feline clone. That honor goes to the multicolored CC (short for Carbon Copy), born in 2001 two days before Christmas Eve. Presented by a Texan researcher, Mark Westhusin, CC was a sensation — even after Dolly the sheep had been cloned in 1996.

So how do you clone a cat? You take a somatic cell from your cat and "starve" it in a low-nutrient broth to reactivate all its genes. This boosted nucleus is then removed and introduced into an enucleated egg cell, also from the original cat. The egg cell now contains a diploid (double) set of chromosomes, just as in normal egg cell fertilization. Electrical impulses are used to stimulate cell division, and once the embryo has reached the eight-cell stage, it can be implanted into the surrogate mother, who gestates the embryo. Hey presto!

But something unexpected happened with CC: her coat pattern was not identical to that of the somatic cell donor, Rainbow. It transpires that the pattern is a result of genetic as well as environmental factors. For example, the position of the embryo in the uterus of the surrogate mother is a deciding factor. Other environmental factors like food intake and health of the surrogate mother can produce minor differences between donor and clone. Besides, only the DNA from the cell nucleus is transferred. This is why existing clones are by no means exact copies of their donors. Little Nicky received, like all animal clones, its donor mother's enucleated egg cell, which represents the cell's "power plant" — the donor's mitochondria with its own genotype.

Where is this heading? The above-mentioned US company will take your cat's tissue for only 295 US dollars. For a basic fee of 1,395 US dollars and an annual

Who Cloned My Cat? Fun Adventures in Biotechnology **by R. Renneberg**
Copyright © 2011 by Pan Stanford Publishing Pte Ltd
www.panstanford.com
978-981-4267-65-6

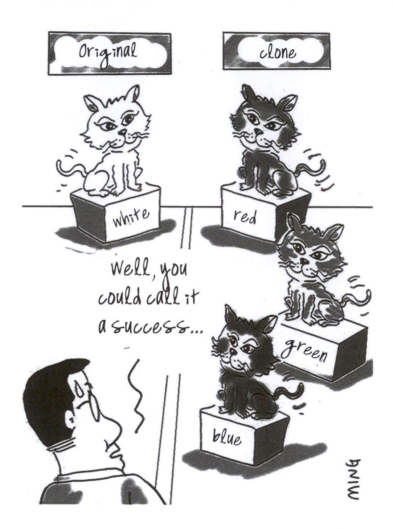

storage fee of 150 US dollars, the cell can be cultivated and stored in liquid nitrogen. Market research has suggested that the maximum customers would be willing to pay for a cloned kitten would be 10,000 US dollars — yet there are already an estimated 10 new customers a day. The company hopes to get cloning projects for 40 cats plus three or four dogs. For 10,000 US dollars rival company Geneticas even promises to deliver a hypoallergenic cloned cat — harmless to those with a cat allergy.

The gender of the donor's cell nucleus is not important, and nucleus and egg cell can come from the same cat. A cat can also be the surrogate mother for its own cell; she can gestate her own clone. A clone of a tomcat will, however, rely entirely on the help of a female — further proof that females can live without males, but men cannot live without women!

For more on this subject, see Chap. 33, *Going to the Dogs?* p. 71 and Chap. 34, *Flipper Gets Artificially Fertilized*, p. 73.

Chapter 27

Even Bacteria Grow Old

"Imagine, ladies and gentlemen, that you are bacteria!" lectured my biology teacher, Dr. Karl Hecht. "You will be undying — not only undyingly in love like you there in the last row! Young man, are you listening!?

Theoretically, bacteria neither age nor die. A single *E. coli* cell can produce two identical copies in 20 minutes, and these copies are able to continue dividing in turn an unlimited number of times."

This idea has been imprinted on my memory until today. But two years ago, I no longer needed to be jealous of bacteria. It was then that researchers at the Biocenter of the University of Basel found that bacteria *do* get old.

Bacteria are prokaryotes, the simplest forms of life, and do not have true cell nuclei. They are assumed to be immortal as long as they are sufficiently nourished and are not exposed to damage from environmental influences. All higher cells on the other hand — eukaryotes — appear to have an expiration date. They fulfill their tasks and divide a few times before they begin to age and finally die.

A prerequisite for aging in bacteria is *asymmetrical* cell division, where the two cells resulting from division are not completely identical. This was observed with the bacterium *Caulobacter crescentus*, which occurs in streams where there is a low level of nutrients. There are two versions of this organism: the flagellated and motile swarmer cells, which are not capable of reproduction, and the non-motile stalk cells, which are able to reproduce. All swarmer cells eventually change into stalk cells, attach to a suitable site, and begin to form swarmer cells again.

Experiments have shown that the ability of stalk cells to reproduce was significantly reduced over a period of about two weeks. Up to 130 offspring were produced, but these did not divide uniformly over that period. Some of the stalk cells had stopped forming swarmer cells by the end of the tests while others only divided sporadically.

It was assumed that the *Caulobacter* under scrutiny did not in any way represent a curiosity in the world of bacteria. What happens, though, when it comes to *symmetrical* cell division?

Who Cloned My Cat? Fun Adventures in Biotechnology by R. Renneberg
Copyright © 2011 by Pan Stanford Publishing Pte Ltd
www.panstanford.com
978-981-4267-65-6

The bacterium *Escherichia coli*, found in the intestine (see also Chap. 25, *Biotech at the Barber's?* p. 53), has long been known for its completely symmetrical division. Does this continuous division make it immortal? Like most bacteria, every 20 minutes or so it separates in the middle to produce two equally sized cell halves. Each new half is then newly synthesized. Each cell consists of an old cell pole inherited from its predecessor and a new pole.

Eric Stewart and his colleagues from the French medical research institute INSERM in Paris followed the fate of dividing bacterial cells depending on the age of their cell poles. In order to do this, they marked individual *E.coli* cells with fluorescent colorant and observed the growth of colonies using an automatic time-lapse microscope. The subsequent evaluation of more than 35,000 cells showed that the bacteria with the oldest cell poles had a lower rate of growth and separation than those with newly synthesized cell halves. Thus, the researchers were convinced that the signs of aging ultimately appear in all organisms.

That I still — despite my age — remember the story about my biology teacher has a simple emotional reason however: I was the young man in the last row.

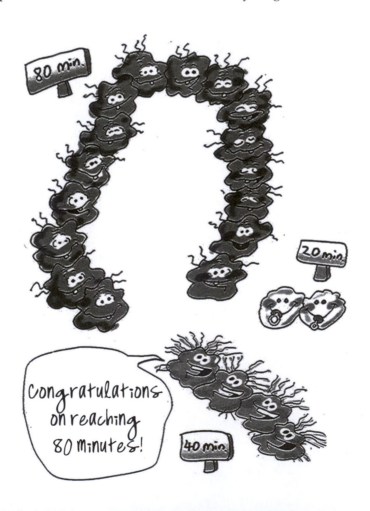

Chapter 28

Give Us This Day Our Daily... Mushroom

Vegetarian? But still longing for that juicy steak? Biotechnology makes your wishes come true!

In the 1960s, it was thought that we were in for severe food shortages in the future as our consumption of protein accelerated. During that time, microorganisms were discovered that could feed not only on sugary food solutions but also on the hydrocarbon-rich components of crude oil, alkanes (paraffins) and methanol.

Eastern Europe, assuming the permanent availability of cheap crude oil, concentrated on alkane-digesting yeasts (*Candida*), while in the West the emphasis was on yeasts and bacteria that use methanol.

Both of these huge projects ended without success. The alkane yeasts were suspected of causing cancer. In the West, the failure of methanol animal feed was caused by European Union subsidies that made skimmed milk powder an unbelievably cheap animal feed additive. Both projects eventually failed on economic grounds as a result of two oil crises. Oil was just too expensive to be converted into protein.

So, a costly fiasco? Well, not really. Biotechnologists garnered inestimable experience in building and operating huge bioreactors.

At the same time, using animal feed turned out to be an unnecessary diversion: the solution can be derived directly from food products. One very successful single-celled product is a mycoprotein ("myco" is from the Greek for fungus) from Rank Hovis McDougall (RHM). The fungus, which can be transformed into passable imitations of fish, poultry and meat, cost the giant foodstuffs producer over 50 million US dollars to develop. The project saw RHM researchers collecting more than 3,000 soil samples from all over the world. As is so often the case, however, the main contender was close by: *Fusarium graminearum* was found near Marlowe in Buckinghamshire, England, and was previously known only for causing root rot in wheat. So, it was a nasty parasite!

Who Cloned My Cat? Fun Adventures in Biotechnology by R. Renneberg
Copyright © 2011 by Pan Stanford Publishing Pte Ltd
www.panstanford.com
978-981-4267-65-6

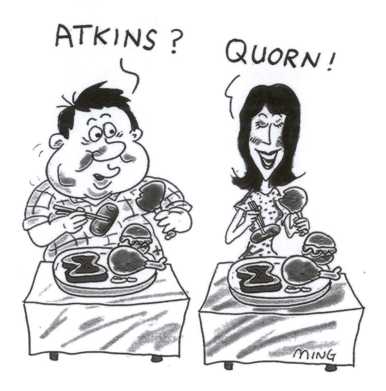

At the time, RHM provided 15 percent of Britain's edible mushroom market. To avoid the anticipated European consumer prejudice against "protein from bacteria," it was stressed from the start that *Fusarium* was a fungus like the mushrooms and truffles that we eat without hesitation.

Aside from the fact that *Fusarium* is virtually odorless and tasteless (making it ideal for meat imitation), its dry weight contains approximately 50 percent protein — a composition similar to grilled steak. The fungus has a lower fat content compared to steak (a mere 13 percent) and this is vegetable fat (ergosterol) with no cholesterol — plus it has a fiber content of 25 percent.

All of this scored points with the increasingly health-conscious public. But the accolades keep on coming. While other microbes contain 15–25 percent of the problematic nucleic acids that can lead to gout, mycoprotein doesn't even contain one percent. The fungus has an amino acid composition recommended by the UN Food and Agriculture Organization (FAO) as "ideal."

Still, the fungus' true trump card is how it can be converted into a full range of imitation food products. According to the length of the fibers, which depends on how long it spends in the bioreactor, the fungus can be used to create anything from soups and biscuits to convincing imitations of poultry, ham or veal.

The nutritional medium for *Fusarium* consists of glucose syrup with ammonia. The syrup can be extracted from any available starch product (such as potatoes, corn or cassava) and the process is much more efficient than the conversion of starch into protein by domestic animals.

In the meantime, the fungus protein was marketed in England as Quorn and has reached the German market as well: Quorn schnitzel, sausages and wieners are for sale. In 1993 big advertising campaigns increased worldwide sales 50-fold to 150 million US dollars.

"My schnitzel tastes a bit like a bioreactor" could soon be the complaint you hear at the German dining table.

Chapter 29

The Moldy Monopoly

The last (not too smart) German emperor William II gave his sailors citric acid to combat scurvy. The result of the kaiser's idea was striking: heavy diarrhea! His majesty was convinced that the acid was the active substance in the fruit. It was excusable back then, given that it was only a symptomatic treatment.

The commercial production of citric acid began under John and Edward Sturge in Selby, England, in 1826. The raw material was the juice of imported Italian citrus fruit (lemons and limes) from which calcium citrate was obtained. This was then easily converted into citric acid.

It was the eminent German chemist Justus von Liebig (1803–1873) who identified the structure of citric acid in 1838, and in 1893, the German microbiologist Carl Wehmer observed that fungi growing on sugar secreted citric acid into the medium. As is so often the case, though, no one read their research articles.

As the demand for citric acid rose after World War I, production from microbes offered a desirable alternative to labor-intensive isolation from expensive imported citrus fruit.

It was an article published in the *Journal of Biological Chemistry* by John N. Currie that was to end Italy's long-held monopoly within a few years. Currie had discovered that *Aspergillus niger* (a mold found on bread) produces far more citric acid than other fungi and he was studying the conditions under which the yields were highest. This time someone read the article. With Currie's help, the Pfizer corporation in New York began the first large-scale production of citric acid in 1923.

During WWI, Italy neglected its citrus plantations, and the price of citric acid soon soared to dizzying heights. Importing countries began to look for cheaper alternatives. In the 1920s, the successful industrial production of citric acid devastated many small farmers in Italy whose livelihoods depended on lemon plantations — an early example of the "collateral damage" caused by the biotech industry.

Microbiologically produced citric acid is chemically identical to citric acid obtained from lemons and is used for flavoring sweets, lemonade, and other foods.

Who Cloned My Cat? Fun Adventures in Biotechnology by R. Renneberg
Copyright © 2011 by Pan Stanford Publishing Pte Ltd
www.panstanford.com
978-981-4267-65-6

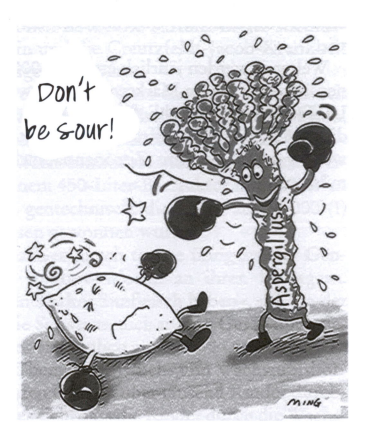

Citric acid is also being considered as an alternative to environmentally harmful polyphosphates in detergents because it forms calcium and magnesium complexes. Because of its ability to bind heavy metals, citric acid is also used as emergency treatment for heavy-metal poisoning. In hospitals, it is used to prevent clotting in blood samples.

Aspergillus niger was cultured on the surface of a liquid medium. Glucose, sucrose, and molasses from sugar beets were the starting substrates.

A hundred years after its foundation, John & E. Sturge (Citric) Ltd., which was based in York, England, adopted Currie's method and combined it with the traditional chemical production of calcium citrate from lemon juice. After WWII, a new submerged biological culture was developed that was easier to control.

Today, bioreactors with capacities of 25,000 to 130,000 gallons (100–500 cubic meters) turn 85 percent of the designated raw material into citric acid. Industrial *Aspergillus* strains remain among the most coveted and guarded possessions in the fermentation industry.

With a world production of 800,000 tons of citric acid every year, even with the best will in the world, it would not be possible to revert to production from citrus fruit — unless every square mile of Italy were covered with lemon trees.

Chapter 30

Finding the Fountain of Youth

Would Napoleon have been an even greater commander if he had received human growth hormone during his childhood? A lack of growth hormone — which is formed in the pea-sized pituitary gland (hypophysis) — leads in extreme cases to stunted growth.

It was not until 1958 that it became possible for children to receive human growth hormone (hGH). At the time, it was taken from the brains of human corpses, a two-year course of treatment for one child requiring 50 to 100 pituitary glands.

After two patients died, however, the sale and use of natural hGH was prohibited at the start of 1985. As the hormone was being isolated, infectious particles from the corpses supposedly contaminated the drug and caused Creutzfeldt–Jakob disease (a degenerative neurological disorder similar to BSE or "mad-cow disease").

Enter the new genetically engineered hGH! The Swedish company Kabi Vitrum, for example (formerly the biggest producer of "natural" human growth hormone in the world), produces hGH from bacteria in a 120-gallon (450-liter) bioreactor in the same quantity that was previously derived from some 60,000 pituitary glands.

The US company Genentech took an unconventional approach to assessing this genetically engineered product: by testing it on its managers. "Managers should have strong muscles for sitting," says Genentech's boss, having had the substance injected into his buttocks. His body tolerated the substance amazingly well, apparently.

In the US, research on dwarfism and hGH has been conducted on over a thousand children. Results indicate that children undergoing growth-hormone therapy grow an average of 2.86 centimeters more per year than children who don't receive growth hormone. For very young kids, the height differences can even reach as much as 4 to 6 centimeters.

Who Cloned My Cat? Fun Adventures in Biotechnology **by R. Renneberg**
Copyright © 2011 by Pan Stanford Publishing Pte Ltd
www.panstanford.com
978-981-4267-65-6

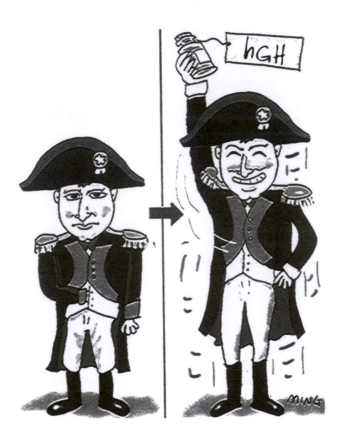

The new findings have resulted in a significant increase in the market for growth hormone. It is notable that bovine growth hormone doesn't just improve milk production in cows, but also has an "anabolic effect": growth hormone increases muscle mass and suppresses the formation of fat — exciting news for bodybuilders and athletes. Growth hormone seems to work effectively in healing wounds and in osteoporosis in the elderly, too. Have we found the biotechnological fountain of youth? In the US, nasal hGH spray is a hit on the "anti-aging" market. But the hGH molecule is too big to be absorbed by nasal stem cells. Don't waste your money on it!

Either way, let's not be too hard on Napoleon — he was by no means a midget. At 1.69 meters he was taller than the average Frenchman of his time. All things are relative. He should probably just have avoided standing beside his towering soldiers all the time.

P.S.: The market for human growth hormone was over 1 billion US dollars in 2007.

Chapter 31

Hong Kong and the Bird Flu

In 1997, as Hong Kong was about to unite with the mainland, bird flu struck. H5N1, the highly pathogenic strain of bird flu, killed on average one in three affected animals. As emergency measures were taken, 1.5 million chickens and ducks were culled in three days — Hong Kong's entire poultry population. Experts believed that the drastic approach taken by then health chief Margaret Chan (see Chap. 65, *From Resignation to WHO*, p. 143) stopped the spread of avian influenza in its tracks.

But the celebrations were premature. The virus was back (or is still present) and there were outbreaks in the middle of December 2003 in Korea, Vietnam, Thailand and Japan, and later in Cambodia, China, Laos and Indonesia. In 2004, 120 million birds were killed. At Japan's and Korea's big farms, it was easier to control the virus by culling, but it proved to be much more difficult to force farmers to kill their flocks in the tiny backyards of Vietnam and Thailand.

But why all the excitement? Specialists warned that the H5N1 bird flu strain could merge with the flu virus in humans or pigs and develop into a deadly "combined" pathogen. Global epidemic strains would result and we'd have a serious pandemic on our hands.

Since 2004, the fatality rate of those infected with H5N1 has risen to 70 percent — compared with "only" 10 percent from SARS (Severe Acute Respiratory Syndrome; see also Chaps. 38, 39 and 48). Between November 2002 and July 2003, there were around 8,000 SARS cases and roughly 800 victims. Although SARS didn't last long, global losses amounted to an estimated 30 to 50 million US dollars, as trade, travel and investment in Asia were disrupted. And the irony was that SARS was not halted by modern medicine or technology but instead through discipline and hygiene.

Only information technology brought real containment — through "teleteaching." I conducted biotech lectures with a camera as my audience; my students stayed at home and used the Internet to follow the classes. (No doubt some dozed off in front of their monitors.) The examination results did not thrill me...

Who Cloned My Cat? Fun Adventures in Biotechnology **by R. Renneberg**
Copyright © 2011 by Pan Stanford Publishing Pte Ltd
www.panstanford.com
978-981-4267-65-6

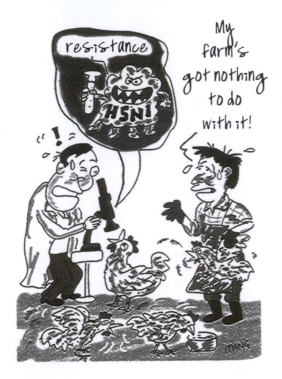

At the same time, multimedia forces sent shock waves through the world. In Hong Kong, the SARS news on TV, on CNN especially, inflated the stories tremendously — and not without a certain malicious glee, it must be said. My poor Mom in Germany could not believe how calm we were in the eye of the typhoon.

In retrospect, the crisis seemed to be largely a result of media overreaction. But there were moments of genuine panic in Hong Kong — like when the residents in one apartment building were quarantined. When the number of infected Chinese nurses rose exponentially in sync with the dramatic rise in newly infected patients — but with a week's delay — even we scientists were restless.

So what is the difference between bird flu and SARS? Influenza viruses of the A-type are more infectious than the SARS coronavirus and their incubation times are shorter. Moreover, the influenza virus can spread before symptoms appear. Measuring an emerging fever, as in the case of SARS, doesn't help much to control the flu.

What is the way forward? In Hong Kong, we've learned a lot from SARS. New biotechnological serums are feverishly under development in China. Novel diagnostic tests will enable speedy influenza testing. Protective masks are at the ready. And 20 million doses of the Tamiflu anti-virus medicine were purchased for Hong Kong in 2005.

Back in 2003, Nobel Prize winner David Baltimore said: "New media technologies are accelerating public anxiety about viruses even faster than new health technologies have enhanced our ability to cope with them. However, credibility is the key to getting things under control."

The clueless Hong Kong leaders who lost face during the SARS incident in 2003 were relieved of their positions two years later. Other countries can also manage that without viruses!

On the subject of the bird flu, see Chap. 38, *Tamiflu Fever in Hong Kong*, p. 81; Chap. 39, *Save the Wild Birds!* p. 83; Chap. 48, *The Cats and the Bird Flu*, p. 101 and Chap. 65, *From Resignation to WHO*, p. 143.

Chapter 32

The Gene Off Switch

Astonishingly, more than 98 percent of our genome has at some point been designated as "junk." This junk DNA does not seem to have any identifiable function. So what is it used for? Another puzzle: humans only have eight times more genes than our bowel bacteria *Escherichia coli*, yet we are considered the "summit of Creation" and our genes are undoubtedly 1,000 times more complex.

A cell nucleus normally contains well-protected double-stranded DNA, which is the template used to synthesize messenger ribonucleic acid (mRNA). The mRNA is single-stranded and carries coding information to the sites of protein synthesis in the cell: the ribosomes. The ribosomes produce proteins according to the RNA template, similar to the DNA. If there are defects in the DNA template (inside the genes), defective mRNA and proteins will be produced as well. This can lead to cancer, for instance.

In 2001, the German scientist Thomas Tuschl from the Max Planck Institute for Biophysical Chemistry in Göttingen found a new approach with the help of short RNA molecules. Using snippets of artificial RNA, he managed to stop the mRNA from working effectively. With this RNA interference (RNAi), mRNA carrying defective messages could be stopped.

The snippets of RNA only need to carry the same sequence as the gene in the cell nucleus DNA that should be made inactive or switched off. The interference snippets trigger the cell's own complex mechanism that destroys the mRNA read from the bad gene. Thus, the messenger on its way to production is stopped by RNAi — and ultimately silenced.

RNAi technology is used to examine the genotype of model organisms and humans for new drug targets. Approximately 5,000 human genes are of interest as drug targets, and it is hoped that they will be found with the aid of RNA snippets known as small interfering RNA (siRNA).

Even siRNA itself can be used as a drug. The list of possible application areas includes rheumatism, Alzheimer's, Parkinson's, cancer, metabolic and auto-immune disorders, and infectious diseases. The idea is that the genes that trigger

Who Cloned My Cat? Fun Adventures in Biotechnology by R. Renneberg
Copyright © 2011 by Pan Stanford Publishing Pte Ltd
www.panstanford.com
978-981-4267-65-6

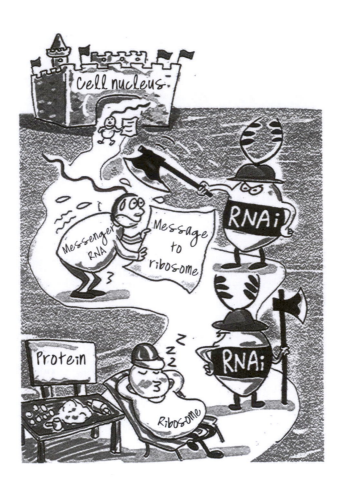

such diseases can be shut down. However, the route from laboratory to clinical application is a long one. Approval of the very first RNAi active substance was granted in 2008.

The greatest difficulty with regard to siRNA treatment is getting the fragile molecules inserted into the cell nuclei where they can be effective. Sensitive material is attacked in the bloodstream and quickly degraded by enzymes.

Are small RNAs and all the genes that are not directly encoding proteins indeed the true rulers in the cell nucleus and responsible for the engine of evolution? What Tuschl achieved artificially has always gone on in nature — it had just been overlooked. Molecular biologists could probably call it their grandest oversight.

P.S.: In 2006, a year after the original publication of this book, American scientists Craig Mello and Andrew Fire won the Noble Prize in Physiology or Medicine for their work investigating the nematode worm *Caenorhabditis elegans*. The worms were injected with RNAi genes that could be switched on and off such that the production of certain proteins was sustained or stopped.

Chapter 33

Going to the Dogs?

Fact: Snuppy (from *Seoul National University* and *puppy*) was the eleventh animal species cloned by humans — after sheep, mice, cows, goats, pigs, rabbits, cats, mules, deer and horses. He was carried to full term by a labrador bitch and looked exactly like his father, an Afghan hound. Snuppy was one lucky dog — the sole survivor among his 1,095 cloned embryo brothers.

Ten years have passed since Dolly the sheep, and "clonology" has not developed as fast as expected — or feared. Mark Westhusin from Texas A&M University, who created CC the kitten (see Chap. 26, *Just as Long as It Catches Mice!* p. 55), gave up trying to clone dogs after three years of experiments. The difficulty with dogs is their egg cells, which leave the ovaries at an early development stage

and mature in the oviduct on their way to the uterus. This makes it hard to determine the right time to extract an egg cell. As with all other cloning, the female nucleus is then removed and replaced with a nucleus from cells taken, in this case, from the ear of an Afghan hound, and this modified egg cell is implanted into the surrogate mother.

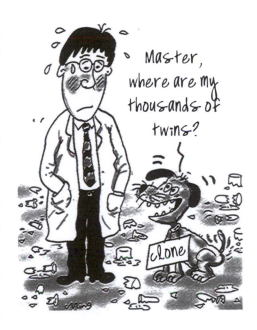

Master, where are my thousands of twins?

clone

Fifteen scientists from South Korea worked for two and a half years on Snuppy, under the strict direction of their star biotechnologist Woo Suk Hwang. He became famous (or notorious if you ask the Pope) the world over as the first to produce human clones — though only for the purpose of obtaining embryonic stem cells. Not long

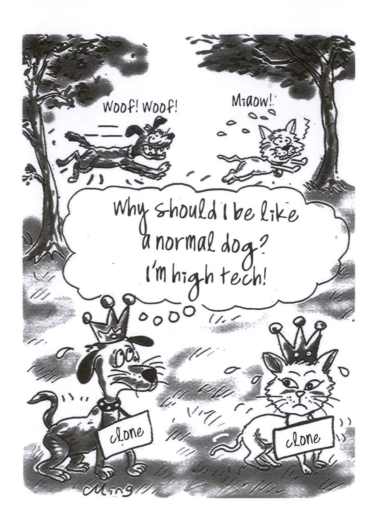

after, scientists were able to repeat the experiments using the genomes of ill patients.

Professor Hwang was flooded with research funding after revealing that he had received an offer from the US (see, however, Chap. 44, *Snuppy, Made in Korea*, p. 93). A Korean postage stamp was even dedicated to him. Hwang has since been disgraced after it was shown that he falsified stem cell data.

In fact, Hwang wanted to breed dog clones as models for human diseases (though that doubtless irritates healthy dog owners), though his rival Mark Westhusin reckons that it was not worth the effort. Still, research on cloned dogs could still be undertaken to find out which genetic and external factors define the characteristic differences among various breeds.

In the meantime, the self-appointed human cloners are going to the dogs. Try explaining who is going to take responsibility for creating thousands of mal-formed embryos from hundreds of surrogate mothers just for the sake of one healthy cloned baby.

Chapter 34

Flipper Gets Artificially Fertilized

Visitors from the Chinese mainland jostle around the baby pool where the dolphins Ada and Gina are doing a show with their offspring Max and Hoi Kei. It's shortly before the opening of Hong Kong Disneyland, and Ocean Park, a marine-themed amusement park in the southern part of Hong Kong Island, is still the number one attraction.

Bottlenose dolphins (*Tursiops truncatus*) are the *de facto* stars — a status they've enjoyed ever since the TV series *Flipper* but even more so now as the public sees how their population is coming under threat from environmental toxins, poor fishing practices and hunting. Now Hong Kong marine biologists and zoologists are attempting artificial insemination in dolphins for the first time. As a curious biotechnology professor, I went there to see for myself.

Artificial insemination in dogs has been around since about 1780. The first German artificial insemination station for cattle was established in 1942. During the 1950s, semen storage methods were developed using liquid nitrogen (–196°C or –321°F), revolutionizing animal breeding. There's certainly a big difference between a hot-tempered bull and a pack of frozen bull semen being shipped across the Atlantic. In industrial countries today, around 90 percent of dairy cows and 60 percent of pigs stem from artificial insemination.

There's no question that the method is very cost efficient: the ejaculate of a stud bull "copulating" with a fake cow yields 400 portions of semen, each containing 20 million spermatozoa. One such bull used for artificial insemination replaces the roughly 1,000 bulls it would require for natural breeding.

Artificial insemination makes it possible to use only the semen of the highest quality breeding stock. In the past 40 years, the performance of dairy cows has increased dramatically — through improved animal feed and without genetic engineering — from 1,000 liters of milk per year to 8,000 liters or more.

It's not just the father that is important in artificial insemination. But even the best breeding cow when inseminated takes nine months to produce a calf — or sometimes two. Nowadays, more progeny can be produced, within the same time period, by injecting the hormone gonadotropin, which initiates superovulation — the maturation of several eggs at the same time. The eggs are then artificially inseminated, and once embryos have developed, they can be taken out quite easily. Up to eight transferable embryos can be obtained in this way and carried by surrogate mothers with a 50 percent success rate. And just like sperm, embryos can be deep-frozen in liquid nitrogen for almost unlimited storage and later implanted into surrogate mothers.

In 1984, the Cincinnati Zoo in Ohio, USA, used Holstein cows as surrogate mothers for a threatened bovine animal, the Malaysian gaur (*Bos gaurus*). In Kenya, oryx (*Taurotragus oryx*), common African antelope, were used as surrogate mothers to rebuild the Bongo antelope population (*Tragelaphus euryceros*). And now the dolphins are having their turn.

Back at Ocean Park, my friend, the talented dolphin trainer Claire Ma, washes her little ones in the pool as they vie for her attention. She's really like a second mother to these lucky little ones. (Read more about her in Chap. 68, *The Chinese also Come from Africa*, p. 149.) I can imagine what they would want most: another copy of their beautiful human mom!

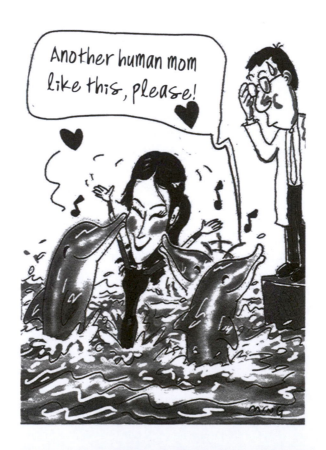

Chapter 35

Heavily Toxic

After Katrina, the disastrous hurricane that hit New Orleans, the after-effects of the catastrophe soon appeared: germs and lead-contaminated water. Lead (Latin: *plumbum*, from *plumbeus* meaning leaden, dull, heavy) is a chemical element, a heavy metal. Our ancestors associated lead with the planet Saturn. Lead, like all heavy metals, blocks enzymes. Among the symptoms of saturnism, or lead poisoning, are paralysis, circulatory problems, joint pain, colic, kidney shrinkage, and deafness. Lead poisoning can also lead to infertility.

Speaking of deafness: Ludwig van Beethoven's (1770–1827) modern fans don't seem to be too bothered by the cause of his deafness. At a Sotheby's auction in London in 1994, four members of the American Beethoven Society acquired a lock of hair from the master, hoping to find an accumulation of mercury. However, they found only a small amount. The minor traces of mercury disproved the much-discussed thesis that Beethoven was suffering from syphilis — a disease once treated with ointments containing mercury. Instead, a large amount of lead was found, and sweetened wine was assumed to be the source of the lead poisoning.

As a constituent of bronze, lead can be found in everything from face powder and paints to drinking cups and frying pans. In ancient Rome, it was used to repair pipes carrying drinking water — which explains where the word "plumber" comes from. Although the Romans were apparently aware of the dangers associated with lead, they overlooked — or ignored — several conspicuous common sources of lead poisoning. One example was keeping vinegar in ceramic pots crafted using lead-containing glazes. The vinegar reacted with the lead and produced lead acetate. This salt of acetic acid is readily soluble in water and has a sweet taste — and is therefore known as lead sugar. The same reaction occurred with sour wine, too. In fact, lead sugar was used as an aphrodisiac. Not even drinking from a golden goblet could have helped: slowly but surely, the Empire poisoned itself.

Some historians believe that, because of saturnism, Julius Caesar (100 BC–44 BC) — despite a series of love affairs — cannot have had more than one son. Caesar Augustus (63 BC–AD 14) was infertile and sexually disinterested. In the

Who Cloned My Cat? Fun Adventures in Biotechnology by R. Renneberg
Copyright © 2011 by Pan Stanford Publishing Pte Ltd
www.panstanford.com
978-981-4267-65-6

first century, most of the aristocrats of the time were sterile. Other Roman emperors Caligula, Nero (who was accused of burning down Rome) and Commodus even suffered from mental disorders that were possibly induced by lead poisoning.

The Roman Empire's famous water pipes that fed most households were essentially made from lead. The lead reacted with the carbon dioxide in the water and gave the pipes a lead carbonate ($PbCO_3$) protective layer. However, some Romans filled their water pipes with wine during festive periods and this layer was removed, creating lead sugar in large quantities. By the Middles Ages, lead sugar was still being used, and even in Beethoven's time it was welcomed by winemakers.

What about today? Well, we filled leaded gasoline into our cars for decades, and we once painted our houses with "white lead" and "red lead" colors — which were most likely used in old buildings in New Orleans, too. Those multicolored ceramic souvenirs we bought on holiday confront us with this substance once again. As far as drinking water goes, here and there, lead pipes can still be found in older houses — in which case it's a good idea to let the water run for a while after it has stayed in the pipes overnight, for example, to flush away any traces of lead.

Wait a minute! I've been engrossed in my book and chewing on my *lead* pencil! But no need to worry: chewing your pencil is a bad habit but it's harmless. Pencils have long been made with graphite (carbon) rather than lead or silver.

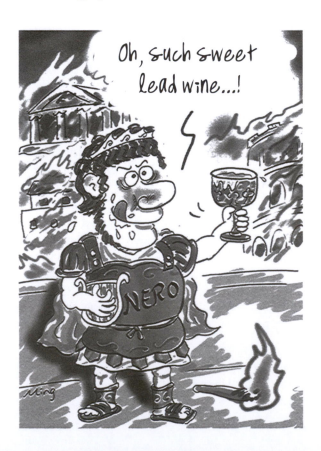

Chapter 36

Smart Medicines

In 1959 when John P. Kane was about to open his new lab at the University of California, he got a phone call that his father had just passed away from a heart attack. The retired general was 66 years old, vegetarian and seemed in good health. The shock catapulted his son into cardiology research. Half a century later, Kane's efforts in the fight against the "world's number one killer" might soon bear fruit.

Kane, together with his wife Mary J. Malloy, has been analyzing the connections between cholesterol and heart attacks for two decades. He started collecting DNA samples in 1985. Now 72, he has analyzed 10,000 genes, about half the human genome. His work has uncovered 20 specific gene variations among people with a tendency toward heart attack. One of those genes, if defective, can lead to higher cholesterol levels in the blood and the liver.

At least half of the genetic variations found, however, have no obvious connection with either cholesterol level or blood pressure. Instead, they are connected to inflammation, which occurs in relation to immune defense. There seem to be different kinds of heart disease — similar to the diversity seen in lung and breast cancers. So rather than an automatic prescription of lipid-lowering medicine, a gene test beforehand would be useful in identifying the type of heart disease — maybe a medicine that inhibits inflammation would turn out to be a better choice.

Welcome to the age of "personalized medicine" — where medications will be individually customized. The era where millions of people take the same medicines for the same ailments will be over. The pharmaceutical industry, for one, isn't exactly thrilled with the prospect: their blockbuster "one-size-fits-all" drugs worth billions might well be relegated to distant second.

There is already proven success with DNA diagnosis: Genentech Inc., for example, developed Herceptin, a successful therapy for 175,000 breast cancer patients that takes into account some genetic variation.

The social impact of this new technology is (as always) controversial. Every year 2.2 million Americans suffer adverse reactions to medication, and some

Who Cloned My Cat? Fun Adventures in Biotechnology by R. Renneberg
Copyright © 2011 by Pan Stanford Publishing Pte Ltd
www.panstanford.com
978-981-4267-65-6

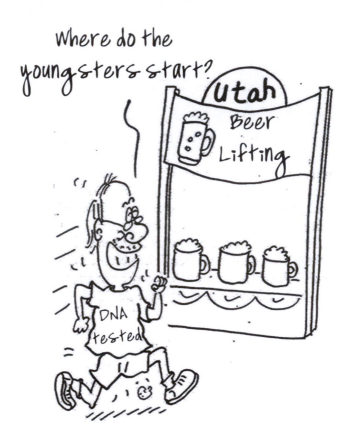

100,000 of those cases are fatal. A simple gene test might have prevented many of those deaths — and saved money in the process. At the same time, however, insurers could reject life or health insurance applications based on the results of such tests. Besides, such testing is expensive: the test for breast or uterine cancer costs around 3,000 US dollars. The big question: Will this lead to medical discrimination? (See Chap. 4, *Expensive and Often Useless*, p. 7.)

So where's the positive side to this story? John Kane has suggested that progress cannot be stopped. A gene test won't bring his father back but it might protect his three grown-up children. They will say of our time that we all lived in the Dark Age of Medicine.

Kane is also comparing DNA samples from his cases with those from healthy elderly patients in order to understand the connection between genes and longevity. Consider the two-week-long Huntsman Senior Games in Utah, where 7000 sportsmen and women compete at bowling, golf, cycling, shooting, mountain biking, racquetball, softball and square dancing — in the age groups of 50, 55, 60, 65 and 70 years old.

Who says all the news from the US is bad? I'm very happy that I'd be eligible to participate as a "young athlete" — in Utah at least. Perhaps in a beer lifting contest?

Chapter 37

Digital Intestinal Bacteria

What do intestinal bacteria do when a cloud of nutritious amino acids approaches? They start their molecular engines! Instead of slow, zigzag movements, they begin twirling in speedy corkscrew-like rotations using their flagella.

Bacteria are fascinating. They are around one thousandth of a millimeter in size and weigh one billionth of a gram. They can move 35 times their body length in a second — that would be like someone swimming at more than 200 kilometers per hour!

Escherichia coli is one of the molecular biologist's pets (along with mice, fruit flies and nematodes; see Chap. 27, *Even Bacteria Grow Old*, p. 57 and Chap. 32, *The Gene Off Switch*, p. 69). It is named after its discoverer, a pediatrician from Vienna called Theodor Escherich (1857–1911). The intestine (Latin: *colon*), where it lives, completes the appellation.

Coli bacteria are important indicators for testing an environment. They colonize our intestines in the billions and — aside from one particular variant that causes serious food poisoning — they are harmless. However, in increased numbers, which is always connected with human or animal excretion, they indicate a lack of hygiene.

Bacterial "engines" are wonders of evolution. They are driven by ATP (adenosine triphosphate, the "fuel" of the cell), and their molecular moving parts rotate at high speed. Their energy essentially comes from the bacteria's food. They're constantly on the lookout for sugars and amino acids — as well as competition from rivals.

A computer program called AgentCell developed at the University of Chicago has simulated how 1000 *E. coli* cells independently move towards a food source. In the simulation, bacteria are located in the middle of a liquid and respond to a chemical stimulator, the amino acid aspartate. In this way, the program explores the behavior of the population of aspartate "lovers" and "loathers" among the *E. coli* cells.

Who Cloned My Cat? Fun Adventures in Biotechnology by R. Renneberg
Copyright © 2011 by Pan Stanford Publishing Pte Ltd
www.panstanford.com
978-981-4267-65-6

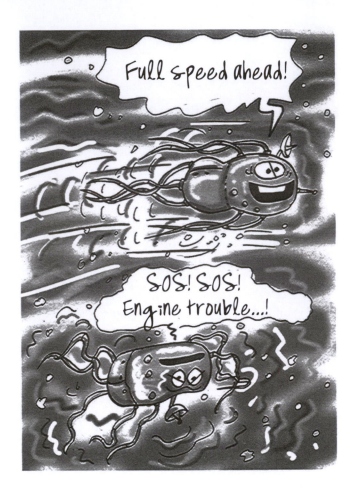

Are such computer bacteria useful — like you might think the corresponding simulated virus would be? Very probably: the next simulation level has shown how bacteria colonize their hosts (our intestines, for example). The short lifespan and reproduction cycle of *E. coli* provide, under ideal conditions, almost five sextillion offspring (five followed by 21 zeros) from each cell in 24 hours.

And there's more about the interesting lives of intestinal bacteria you should know. For example, they are capable of transferring DNA to their partners through so-called sex pili, nano-sized pipe-like appendages similar in construction to flagella. This is how bacteria share resistant genes. For example, the ability to produce enzymes that render antibiotics ineffective can be passed on — a headache that causes big problems for our current therapeutic methods.

DNA exchange takes about half an hour on average. But these beasties have an average lifespan of just 20 minutes. So when they "have sex," it takes them longer than an entire lifetime! As Gunter Stent, one of the pioneers of gene technology, put it: "Bacteria, you have it better!"

Chapter 38

Tamiflu Fever in Hong Kong

Bird Garden, the wonderful bird market in Yuen Po Street in Hong Kong, is losing visitors, and thousands of songbirds wait for new owners in vain. The city has fallen under the spell of the bird flu and the H5N1 virus. Meanwhile, the trade in live chickens and ducks is as vibrant as ever. "There's no reason to panic!" says the government — reason enough for skeptical Hong Kongers to believe the opposite.

Newspaper headlines like FLU MEDICINE ALMOST SOLD OUT only exacerbate the situation. The wonder drug they're talking about is Tamiflu® from Swiss pharmaceutical giant Rocher. Its active substance, oseltamivir, blocks the virus enzyme neuraminidase: newly established viruses are prevented from leaving the affected cell and attacking healthy ones.

"Yet where there is danger, a rescuing element grows as well," wrote the German poet Friedrich Hölderlin. Indeed, the bird flu originated in Asia but it is also where they discovered an herbal remedy. You can find *bajiao*, or star anise, in every Chinese kitchen. It is obtained from an oily, eight-pointed star-shaped fruit from the small evergreen *shikimi* tree (*Illicium verum*), a distant relative of the magnolia, which grows in south China. In Asia it has enjoyed a long history as a cure for stomach ache, toothache and lack of virility. And, naturally, it is used as a spice as well — ironically enough, for duck-based dishes. In Germany, in the form of an essential oil, it turns up in Christmas cookies and gingerbread cakes.

These days, the shikimic acid from star anise is the star ingredient in Tamiflu®. Each ton of oseltamivir provides a million packs, each containing ten pills. This quantity of Tamiflu® is sufficient to supply 100 to 200 million people for five days. But demand has skyrocketed to such extent that Roche will have to produce Tamiflu® until 2007 just to fulfill current advance orders from 40 countries — even after production capacity has been doubled. After hurricane Katrina, Americans are only now waking up to the dangers — with three billion dollars ready to spend on Tamiflu®. But they'll have to get in line after Romania and Hungary! It will be interesting to see how things turn out.

Who Cloned My Cat? Fun Adventures in Biotechnology **by R. Renneberg**
Copyright © 2011 by Pan Stanford Publishing Pte Ltd
www.panstanford.com
978-981-4267-65-6

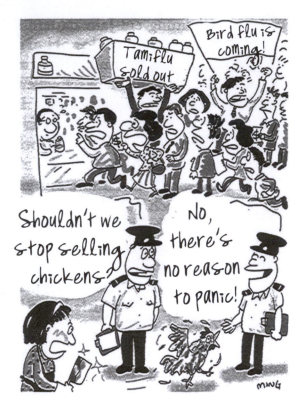

Various countries have tried pressuring Roche into licensing the production of Tamiflu® for free. But it's been a long and futile road. Meanwhile, Thailand and Taiwan have both expressed their desire to produce of a generic version. Roche seems to be making nice. And why not? Star anise harvesting falls between March and May, and Roche has already bought up almost 90 percent of the feedstock. Given that processing takes a whole year, their competitors won't stand a chance.

Since we are working on a rapid virus test in Hong Kong, a joint effort with a small company in Berlin-Buch, I needed Tamiflu® for myself — just in case. Clutching a prescription from the university hospital, I went to the nearest pharmacy. The handwritten note on the door seemed like bad news, but all I could understand was the word "Tamiflu."

As someone who has lived in former East Germany, though, I know the tricks and I played dumb. I went straight to the head pharmacist, who was very easy to spot on account of his advanced age, gold-rimmed specs and semi-bald head. "My dear colleague," I said with a sigh. "We need your valuable scientific assistance!" He bowed three times and replied loudly, "Sorry, no Tamiflu! You wait!" Then he scribbled three Chinese characters on my prescription and whispered, "One thousand!" I shoved two 500 Hong Kong dollar bills quickly into his hand.

I suddenly felt like I was in a time machine: back in East Berlin 25 years ago, in a butcher's shop in Florastrasse in Pankow, a regular customer would pay blindly and get a mysterious package in return. The package would be opened outside the shop — "Aha! Beef fillet!" Hong Kong, October 25, 2005: I open the package outside the shop. "Aha! Five packs of Tamiflu!"

Find out more on this subject in Chap. 31, *Hong Kong and the Bird Flu*, p. 67; Chap. 39, *Save the Wild Birds!* p. 83; Chap. 48, *The Cats and the Bird Flu*, p. 101 and Chap. 65, *From Resignation to WHO*, p. 143.

Chapter 39

Save the Wild Birds!

Getting caught feeding pigeons or other wild birds in Hong Kong gets you a fine of 1,500 Hong Kong dollars (about 200 US dollars). Alternatively, you'll get five minus points — 16 of those and you could lose your affordable little housing unit.

Personally, I keep nine inseparable Dwarf fig-parrots in my apartment — and a Hill myna, which often brawls outside in the garden (in a cage of course). Fortunately for me, I live in a residence that belongs to the university and I can get away with it. As it happens, I am currently working on a rapid virus test with a company from Berlin.

Bird lovers in Hong Kong have traditionally been ignored or even ridiculed — until now. But all of a sudden *everyone* seems interested in our opinion: Are sparrows and wild pigeons dangerous?

The *Hong Kong Bird Hotline* is a heritage from traditional British bird lovers. It was from them that I heard about the arrival of three Black-faced spoonbills at the Mai Po Marshes. As I got there, hundreds of ornithologists were already pointing their telephoto lenses in the direction of the star birds. Around April–May and September–October, millions of migrating birds visit this nature reserve in the northwest. The wetland area is an important stopover for the exhausting flight of around 16,000 kilometers, but it's also home to a shrimp-farming business that supplies Hong Kong's restaurants. Will this become another influenza hotspot?

Since I'm only a hobby ornithologist, I consulted the head of the ornithological institute in Radolfzell, Dr. Wolfgang Fiedler, about the matter. Aquatic poultry is indeed a reservoir for influenza viruses, but the original bird flu virus has rarely had much affect on them — even when they become infected. It is only after the virus is transferred to domestic poultry that it transforms into a highly pathogenic bird flu virus (HPAI virus).

The current outbreak can be traced back to the HPAI virus, H5N1, which, it is presumed, emerged in domestic ducks in south China at the end of the 1990s. All patients infected with H5N1 had close contact with infected chickens, ducks or

Who Cloned My Cat? Fun Adventures in Biotechnology by R. Renneberg
Copyright © 2011 by Pan Stanford Publishing Pte Ltd
www.panstanford.com
978-981-4267-65-6

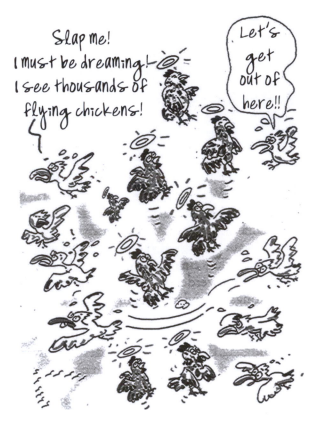

Slap me!
I must be dreaming!
I see thousands of
flying chickens!

Let's get out of here!!

pigs — either on a farm or on a plate. Whether there is a possibility of human-to-human transmission is still the subject of much controversy.

Could migrating birds really be responsible for the long-haul transport of the HPAI virus? The spatial and temporal patterns of HPAI outbreaks don't really match bird migration patterns. In any case, ornithologists doubt that birds infected with the H5N1 virus are physically capable of flying long distances. So far, there hasn't been a single case where the H5N1 virus has been isolated from a clinically healthy wild bird. The sick wild birds that have been reported have in most cases been infected through contact with domestic poultry.

Two cases out of three of the virus being introduced into countries in the EU were as a result of human transportation: smuggled hawk eagles and parrots were kept in the same quarantine station as birds from the Far East. The bottom line is: we should actually be protecting wild birds from domestic poultry!

I remember clearly my younger days living in the former East Germany when the Alfred Hitchcock movie "The Birds" was showing on TV. The next morning, the sparrows, tits and crows in my small village got wary looks. "And we feed these mean creatures every day!" said our neighbor, revealing himself as a watcher of West German TV.

Read more on this subject in Chap. 31, *Hong Kong and the Bird Flu*, p. 67; Chap. 38, *Tamiflu Fever in Hong Kong*, p. 81; Chap. 48, *The Cats and the Bird Flu*, p. 101; and Chap. 65, *From Resignation to WHO*, p. 143.

Chapter 40

Depression from Antidepressants?

"Are you depressed? Don't worry, it is only because your neurotransmitter, serotonin, is unbalanced!" trumpets the US pharmaceutical industry in its million-dollar campaigns. In the US, expensive drugs called selective serotonin reuptake inhibitors (SSRIs) can be sold directly to patients. In 2004, just one of these drugs made a three million US dollar profit.

How can the effects of antidepressants be made clear to customers? Serotonin is transferred from one cell to another as a neurotransmitter. These neurotransmitters cross the gaps between cells. The receptor cell receives part of the serotonin and returns a small part of it back to the submitter cell — like two people having a conversation. In a depressed patient, the first nerve cell receives too much serotonin in return, the result being that a third nerve cell receives too little. It's as if two people are engrossed in conversation and a third can't get a word in — an unbalanced conversation resulting in depression! You can see it on any talk show on TV: the non-stop talker always has to be reigned in. SSRIs do exactly that: they play the role of the talk show host. Simple, right?

Well, yes, but there's just one snag. In the open-access journal *PLoS* (Public Library of Science) *Medicine*, Jonathan Leo (Lake Erie College of Osteopathic Medicine in Bradenton, Florida) and Jeffrey Lacasse (Florida State College of Social Work) have sharply criticized the misleading advertisements of SSRIs.

The science journal *Nature* agrees: such drugs might have helped some but they also have adverse effects. In the rival journal *Science*, scientists from Columbia University have reported that animals given SSRI antidepressants at a young age show similar symptoms to animals with genetically related defective serotonin transport.

Leo and Lacasse have argued that the mechanisms through which these drugs are meant to work aren't obvious. For instance, it has never been verifiably proven that depression is caused by a lack of serotonin. Surely, our brains aren't really that simple. Bettina Reiter, a psychiatrist from Vienna, says, "It is beyond doubt that neurotransmitters play a part in controlling the emotions, but the relationships are significantly more complex."

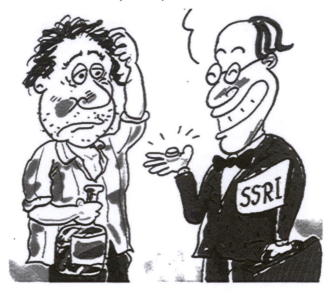

Before I tell you the price, here's a pink pill for free!

The logical explanation is also too simplistic: aspirin generally cures headaches, but headaches aren't caused by a lack of aspirin. Also, some experiments involving sports activities have shown how placebos for depression gave the same or even better results.

Bettina Reiter also points this out: people tend not to deal with the root causes of depression but instead take an antidepressant to alter mood.

In his book *Brave New World*, Aldous Huxley had a frightening vision: the perfect, side-effect-free antidepressant, *soma*, available to all. In the book, you can read: "… there is always soma, delicious soma, half a gramme for a half-holiday, a gramme for a week-end, two grammes for a trip to the gorgeous East, three for a dark eternity on the moon…"

Here in Hong Kong, I have a home remedy for my German depression: the TV remote control. When our irritating politicians appear on Deutsche Welle, I just switch channels! I don't want to be part of some serotonin reuptake inhibitor experiment.

Chapter 41

Mussel Extract Takes On Vioxx®

From tennis elbow through joint wear and tear from aging to rheumatic inflammation — it seems almost everyone has joint problems these days. In Germany, studies suggest that every second person does.

Thus, the arrival of the cyclooxygenase (COX) inhibitor on the market in 1999 couldn't have been more timely: by inhibiting cyclooxygenase, the pain signals that are caused by inflammation can be blocked. The relief for arthritis patients was substantial. But it came at a price — indeed, it was a roaring trade for some. In the first year after its debut, the "miracle drugs" celecoxib (Celebrex®) and rofecoxib (Vioxx®) were prescribed about 100 million times. Celebrex® ranks sixth on the pharmaceutical best-seller list, with a 3.3 billion US dollar profit.

In principle, the new drugs should only affect COX enzymes, but there were strong suspicions that Vioxx® was the cause of deadly heart attacks since it hit the market. Some 140,000 cases were reported in the US alone. The British medical journal *The Lancet* published related research by one expert, David Graham, on the Internet — against the will of his employer, the US Food and Drug Administration. The study found that patients who took Vioxx®, compared to fellow sufferers on other drugs, had a one-third higher risk of developing acute heart disease. Vioxx® manufacturer Merck was soon forced to withdraw the drug from the market.

Celebrex®, from the top pharmaceutical manufacturer Pfizer, is coming under the same kind of scrutiny. Pfizer has begun clinical research that should be complete by 2010.

Professor Georges Halpern (see Chap. 60, *Another Spoonful of Red Wine?* p. 133), a California scientist with French roots who teaches at the Hong Kong Polytechnic University, foresaw all of these problems. He has blatantly labeled the big pharmaceutical companies greedy and unscrupulous criminals, claiming that research results were falsified and money that should have been spent on assessing risks was instead used for advertising. He believes that the pharmaceutical multinationals should be sued for millions — just like Big Tobacco.

Who Cloned My Cat? Fun Adventures in Biotechnology by R. Renneberg
Copyright © 2011 by Pan Stanford Publishing Pte Ltd
www.panstanford.com
978-981-4267-65-6

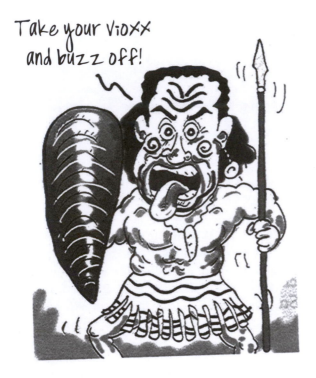

Take your Vioxx
and buzz off!

Besides, there are low-cost alternatives! Halpern mentions sport for example, particularly swimming. Using the painkiller "classics" acetaminophen (paracetamol) and aspirin (see Chap. 22, *One Pill for (Almost) Everything?* p. 47) is another possibility, but, of course, they are produced cheaply in China and India so there is no profit for the pharmaceutical giants.

Nature offers more help — in the form of the green-lipped mussel (*Perna canaliculus*). Observations of the lifestyles of the native coastal dwellers of New Zealand, where these mussels are endemic, have demonstrated an absence of rheumatic disease. These Maori enjoy life into old age without joint problems — unlike their relatives inland — thanks to their large mussel consumption.

The connection between mussels and rheumatism has, in fact, been scientifically verified. The green-lipped mussel contains glucosaminoglycans and amino sugar, primary components of joint lubricant, as well as orthosilicic acid (which strengthens bones and tissues) and omega-3 and omega-6 fatty acids (which inhibit inflammation).

Green-lipped mussels are now cultivated on the coasts of New Zealand. It takes them two years to attain full maturity. The plankton that they feed on have developed a mechanism to protect themselves from ultraviolet light (which also triggers inflammation) and this is passed on to the mussels. The name of the oil extracted from the mussels is lypirol, which works effectively for rheumatic joint problems accompanied by severe inflammation. It's easy to see why Georges Halpern calls his new book *The Inflammation Revolution*.

It seems no matter where you look, inflammation is everywhere. Or is that *inflation*? Well, that too, of course!

Chapter 42

Clone Trees That Glow in the Dark

Finding the perfect Christmas tree was a real headache back in the former East Germany. Some would come home without much more than a branch. Nowadays, money is all it takes to solve the problem.

The origin of the Christmas tree tradition is a bit of a mystery. Evergreen plants symbolize vitality; one might think that decorating the house with green plants will bring its occupants good health. At the turn of the year, the Romans would decorate their houses with laurel wreaths. In northern Europe, people once hung fir branches in early winter to keep bad spirits away. The first mention of a Christmas tree is from 1419: bakeries in Freiburg, Germany had a tree variously decorated with sweets and cookies — that children were allowed to plunder after New Year.

There are huge farms specializing in the cultivation of Christmas trees, and each year in the US and Canada alone around 40 million are harvested. Farmers attempt to achieve the perfect shape by trimming. Trees must have straight trunks, and a nice conical shape, with branches angled at 45 degrees and thick, strong needles. But only one in 10,000 trees is perfect.

Surely this a case that can be solved with biotechnology. Enter the clones! In fact, scientists from Michigan State University are already working on the Douglas fir and Scots pine. Their new trees should grow faster and be resistant to fungus and insects. There should also be an increase in the utilization rate from 60–70 to 95 percent as well as a reduction in the need for pesticides.

Denmark, the world's champion exporter of Christmas trees, has been experimenting since 1999. Around 10 million trees are exported every year (Nordmann fir almost exclusively), but almost the same number goes to waste due to growth defects — a considerable expense.

At the Botanic Institute of the University of Copenhagen, scientists divide the tiny seeds into two and freeze one of them at –196 degrees Celsius (liquid nitrogen). The other is planted in a culture medium and placed in a sterile incubator. After four months, the seedling, which has grown to about 2.5 centimeters in size, is transferred to greenhouses in Funen Island. "In five or six years, we will see

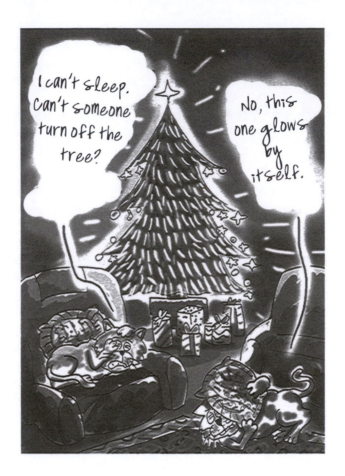

how these trees have developed, and we can then select the ones with the best genetic quality," says Dr. Jens Find. When the perfect tree is found, its frozen counterpart will then be used to create thousands or millions of copies. Whether people can appreciate a forest of identical trees remains to be seen.

Does it get any better than this? Of course! How about a tree that glows without candles! With the gene from the firefly enzyme luciferase, it's already been possible to make tobacco plants glow. Why not do the same with fir trees? You'll just have to water your Christmas tree with luciferin. You could also use the green fluorescent protein (GFP) from the *Aequorea* jellyfish, which glows by itself — though only under UV light. What if we somehow combine luciferase and GFP to avoid the need for UV light? Special water will still be needed say researchers. Besides, it would be nice to be able to switch the tree lights on and off, wouldn't it?

Picture the distressed father on the Christmas Eve of the future, shouting, "For God's sake! Where's the luciferin? Our neighbor's tree is already on!"

Happy holidays!

More on glowing organisms can be found in Chap. 10, *Glow, Little Fish, Glow!* p. 19.

Chapter 43

A Brief History of Ecstasy

The role of drug inventor wasn't always played by our present-day drug laboratories. In the Germany of the past, scientific discovery was driven by the enthusiasms of the associates of the emperor — Kaiser Wilhelm II.

Amphetamine, for instance, a chemical derivative of benzene, was first synthesized in Berlin as far back as 1887. Initially, it was used as a decongestant but its stimulating effects soon became apparent. Later, it would keep WWII pilots awake and help soldiers control stress on the battlefield. Amphetamine was still available for sale after the war, especially in Japan. In the 1950s, about two million people were using amphetamine to combat physical fatigue.

One of the synthetic derivatives of amphetamine, which was discovered in 1891–92, is 3,4-methylenedioxy-N-methamphetamine (MDMA) — better known today as ecstasy. At the time, the Darmstadt-based pharmaceutical company E. Merck was producing and selling morphine (since 1827) and cocaine (since 1884); their addictive effects were only understood later.

MDMA seemed to have no useful medical purpose, but as an intermediate compound in the preparation of another substance, its production was patented in 1912. It wasn't until the early 1950s that the US army and the Central Intelligence Agency (CIA) began to take an interest in MDMA, calling it "the truth drug" (code-named EA-1475). Although test subjects were astonishingly candid about their experiences under the influence of ecstasy, the drug officially returned to the shelves again.

The American chemist Alexander Schulgin (born in 1925) made a breakthrough in 1976 when he discovered a new method of synthesizing MDMA. His first experiences working with mescaline (a drug derived from the Peyote cactus) led to his becoming a drug inventor.

Ecstasy intensifies the distribution of two neurotransmitters in the brain: dopamine (associated with feelings of pleasure) and noradrenalin, both of which work against the sleep-inducing serotonin. A person who takes ecstasy is thus wide awake and experiences pleasant, mild hallucinations.

Who Cloned My Cat? Fun Adventures in Biotechnology **by R. Renneberg**
Copyright © 2011 by Pan Stanford Publishing Pte Ltd
www.panstanford.com
978-981-4267-65-6

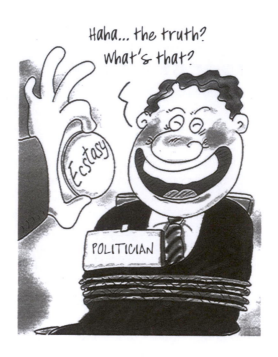

Shulgin synthesized hundreds of psychoactive chemicals — and tried them out on himself. For a long time, he had a license from the state to work with illegal substances. Leo Zeff, a psychiatrist from Oakland, popularized ecstasy among the 1970s psychotherapeutic community, paving the way for its more widespread use. By the early 1990s, the drug had traveled via England back to its place of birth in the Kaiser's homeland.

The debate about ecstasy's effects on health is still raging. Laboratory rats have been found to suffer long-term damage to brain cells — after just one dose of MDMA. The drug has also caused havoc because it increases body temperature: hot, sweaty parties and ecstasy are a deadly combination. No wonder the substance joined the list of illicit drugs in 1985. Once a useless compound produced by the chemists of the Kaiser's Germany, MDMA has evolved into the party drug of choice — often with devastating effects.

Personally, I find the notion of using MDMA as a "truth drug" most interesting. Television stations could get top politicians on their talk shows — especially during election time — and serve them MDMA cocktails. "Welcome to another exciting round of your favorite show, folks: 'TELLING THE TRUTH WITH ECSTASY'!"

Oh, I should patent the idea right away!

Chapter 44

Snuppy, Made in Korea

Snuppy is real — that much, it seems, we know after the institute HumanPass Inc. revealed the identity of the Korean cloned dog to the world. Kim Minkyu of the veterinary clinic of Seoul National University (SNU), who created Snuppy with Hwang Woo-Suk, summed it up thus: "The dog was cloned as follows: a cell nucleus is removed from the egg cell and replaced with nuclei from the body cell of the Afghan hound to be cloned." His team informed the British scientific journal *Nature* that both DNA and mitochondria analyses — which are used to verify successful cloning — were carried out.

Hwang's research team published their groundbreaking work in *Nature* on August 4, 2005. However, the authenticity of the cloned Afghan hound was thrown into question after it was discovered that later work by the same team involving the creation of human embryonic stem-cell lines was, in large part, fabricated.

When I met Hwang myself, my impression was only of a tireless scientist. My Korean colleagues here at the university don't condemn him outright — but instead talk of the affair as if it were a Greek tragedy. A farmer's son, Hwang had become world famous despite his humble beginnings and had, for a time, given the divided Koreas a new self-confidence.

The falsifications relating to his stem-cell work were so clumsy, however,

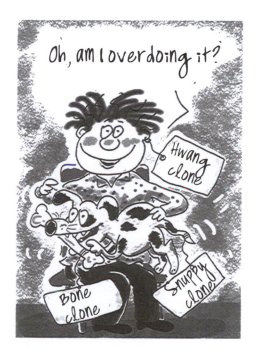

Who Cloned My Cat? Fun Adventures in Biotechnology by R. Renneberg
Copyright © 2011 by Pan Stanford Publishing Pte Ltd
www.panstanford.com
978-981-4267-65-6

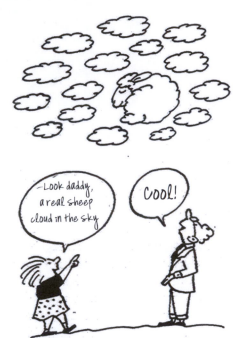

that Hwang labeled it a conspiracy, claiming that cells were deliberately switched. Is it possible that his co-workers "tweaked" their beloved boss' results? What is true is that some cell cultures were destroyed by infection in early 2005 and his team was under a lot of pressure to produce results.

Hwang was adamant that his research group possessed the cloning technologies as described. According to SNU, five human stem-cell cultures were developed in Hwang's laboratory — and they were indeed cloned. However, they were at an early stage of development and were in fact created *after* the publication in *Science* in May 2005.

"*Nature* will bring the investigation into the details of the publication [regarding Snuppy] to a conclusion," said Katherine Mansell, a representative for the magazine. New findings are being nervously awaited in *Science* editorial departments as well. The two most renowned scientific publishers in the world are under fire. The editors of *Science* in Washington should ask themselves whether their overeager publishing politics drove them to pounce on such clumsily falsified work. *Nature*, on the other hand, will just be lucky if Snuppy is proved to be a real clone — given the important information that was lacking from their published article.

Meanwhile, the investigating commission from SNU is conducting tests at a second institute — since HumanPass Inc. was actually commissioned by Hwang himself. The results are pending.

So where does the boss' brazen attitude come from? This is what my Korean friends jokingly say: "The real Hwang is sitting with his feet up at home while his clone apologizes on TV!"

For more on this subject, see Chap. 26, *Just as Long as It Catches Mice!* p. 55 and Chap. 33, *Going to the Dogs?* p. 71.

Chapter 45

Molecular Laundresses

Have you ever seen enzymes at work with your own eyes? No? Are you sure? Because everyone has watched how fast wounds heal (from clotting enzymes) or how cuts in apples, potatoes or bananas turn brown (from the enzyme phenoloxidase).

We also use industrially produced enzymes to wash our laundry. Anyone who has a baby knows how hard it is to wash out stains containing protein like milk, egg yolk, blood or cocoa. Protein is difficult to dissolve solely with water; it coagulates at high temperature and stays even more stubbornly in fabrics.

Clothing stains are a combination of dust, soot and organic substances. Dirt stays especially on bedding and garments because of the fats and proteins left by the body: they work on the dirt like an adhesive. During washing, fatty dirt is dissolved by surface-active substances (detergents), separating it from the fabric.

At the beginning of the 20th century, Otto Röhm (1876–1939) from Darmstadt in Germany had the idea of washing fabrics with a diluted extract from the pancreas. By 1914, his company was producing a laundry agent call Burnus® containing pancreatic protease from pigs. It was a good enough idea, but the product wasn't successful because pancreatic enzymes were quite expensive and not sufficiently stable in alkaline washing soda.

Things didn't change until 1959 when the enzyme subtilisin, a protease that also works in soapsuds, was isolated from the bacteria *Bacillus licheniformis*. Today, between about 200 to 500 milligrams of this alkaline protease per kilogram is added to detergent. These enzymes will "eat" anything. All kinds of adhesive proteins are broken down, leaving laundry clean "to the pores."

Enzyme-based detergents had their glory days in the mid-1960s in the US and Western Europe. But by 1970 they had come under a hail of criticism as enzymatic dust was shown to be causing allergic reactions among production workers. The problem was solved by granulating the detergent powders. These days supermarkets sell various forms, including wax-coated granules, tabs or liquid detergent.

Who Cloned My Cat? Fun Adventures in Biotechnology by R. Renneberg
Copyright © 2011 by Pan Stanford Publishing Pte Ltd
www.panstanford.com
978-981-4267-65-6

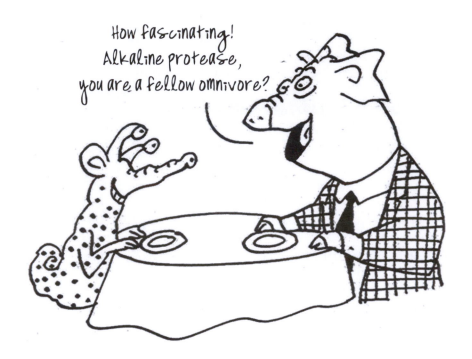

How fascinating! Alkaline protease, you are a fellow omnivore?

In the meantime, manufacturers are adding not only protease but also amylase in order to dissolve starch as well as lipase to dissolve grease. Another quality of bio-detergent has become significant too: since the enzymes work optimally between 50–60 degrees Celsius, boiling is no longer necessary and energy can be saved.

We've just been celebrating Chinese New Year — always a good excuse for a lavish dinner with friends. Proving that us "long noses" are unskilled with chopsticks, my spring roll took a tumble into the tasty sauce, and — *plop!* — I got a big brown spot on my new white shirt. It was funny for the Chinese, of course. They lifted their glasses and toasted the wonderful Chinese cuisine!

The shirt was saved later: half an hour soaking in lukewarm water with enzymatic detergent and the ugly stain was gone. Here's to you, amylase, protease and lipase! Cheers!

For more on this subject, read Chap. 12, *"Irashaimase, Baioteku"*, p. 25 and Chap. 74, *Genetic Engineering in Your Washer*, p. 163.

Chapter 46

My Own Private Genome?

Suppose I went to a laboratory, put my blood sample on the table, and asked for my DNA sequence. How much would it cost me? There are about 3,400,000,000 base pairs (the DNA components A, T, C, G) spread across 23 chromosomes pairs. That's quite a lot of data — once calculated to be equivalent to the information in 200 New York telephone books with 1000 pages each!

American human genome hunter J. Craig Venter, who successfully competed with the government's research labs (see Chap. 3, *The Little Roaring Mouse*, p. 5 and Chap. 77, *DNA Gunshots into the Sea*, p. 169), has offered a reward of 10 million US dollars to the team that invents a method of delivering — for 1000 US dollars — a complete human DNA sequence.

Has anyone even come close to winning the millions? Recently, the US magazine *The Scientist* compared prices. A standard system from Applied Biosystems costs about 365,000 US dollars and can analyze 2.8 million base pairs in chronological order per day. That seems fast, but it would take 2100 days (almost six years) to uncover my complete genome. That's too long for the Harvard Professor George Church, who says, "In some emergency situations, DNA sequences are needed almost immediately!" Another genome analysis laboratory wants the impressive sum of 11 million US dollars for the work.

What about the new sequencer from 454 Life Sciences? The Genome Sequence 20 (priced at 500,000 US dollars) doesn't use the traditional method and analyzes 40 million base pairs in just four hours. Quite a dramatic improvement! I could get my result in less than a month, though it would still cost me about 900,000 US dollars.

But now the experts are saying that the genome cannot be determined correctly with only one round of sequencing — at least 8–15 rounds are required! That means I'll have to cough up 7–14 million. And I'll have to wait for a year.

This year Solexa intends to hit the one billion base pair mark in two days. For 100,000 US dollars, 30 repeated measurements should be possible. Helicos Biosciences tops the list with 125 million base pairs per hour — 7.5 billion a day. That corresponds to the genomes of six people every day with ten-fold repetition!

Who Cloned My Cat? Fun Adventures in Biotechnology by R. Renneberg
Copyright © 2011 by Pan Stanford Publishing Pte Ltd
www.panstanford.com
978-981-4267-65-6

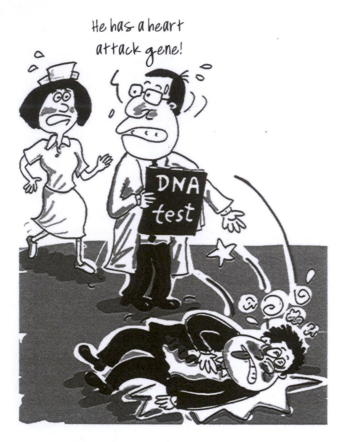

He has a heart attack gene!

In the meantime, Professor Church has started his own "Personal Genome Project." His plan is to ask 100 "well-informed" volunteers for their approval to make their genome sequences with all their available medical results freely accessible on the Internet. He hopes to make a valuable comparison between genotypes and phenotypes.

Of course, incorrigibly enthusiastic about progress as I am, I leapt at the chance to take part in the project. My Chinese co-workers wisely put a damper on my eagerness: "So you want to entrust your data to the Bush administration? You, who work for the Hong Kong government?"

"Well, no, that wasn't my intention, but…"

"Okay, but then your Hong Kong life insurance company can find out from the Internet when you'll be getting a heart attack and promptly raise your premium!"

"Oh yes! You are so right. Thank you!"

Professor Church has a grand total of three potential approvals so far — and they're all still pending.

Read more on this subject in Chap. 67, *DNA and My Ancestors*, p. 147 and Chap. 68, *The Chinese also Come from Africa*, p. 149.

Chapter 47

Goethe and the Caffeine

"Ah, how sweet coffee tastes — lovelier than a thousand kisses!" For over two decades, the famous German composer Johann Sebastian Bach (1685–1750) visited Zimmerman's Coffee House in Leipzig twice a week. His "Coffee Cantata," based on the writings of Christian Friedrich Henrici, just goes to prove the enduring allure of caffeine.

It took some 90 years before this famous pick-me-up was chemically isolated. In fact, over 60 kinds of plants produce caffeine, apparently to protect themselves against insects. The famous German poet Johann Wolfgang von Goethe (1749–1832) is believed to have contributed to the discovery of this most popular of natural products.

Friedlieb Ferdinand Runge, a young chemistry student from Göttingen, went to visit Jena University (in central Germany). There he met Goethe's right-hand man, the chemist Johann Wolfgang Döbereiner (1780–1849), from whom he learned analytical chemistry. Runge was born in 1794 near Hamburg and studied pharmacy before leaving his hometown in 1816 for Berlin, Jena and Göttingen to study medicine. When he met Döbereiner in Jena, he had already had experience in the chemical study of poisonous and medicinal plants.

Döbereiner was so impressed with Runge's experiments on cat's eyes that he said, "You are very important, and this evening I will tell Goethe about you." That was how the great privy councilor Goethe had "condescended to grant an audience to an insignificant student with a cat under his arm," as Runge later wrote.

Goethe was interested in the physiology of the eye because of his own studies on the theory of colors. Thus, one morning in 1819, the young scientist demonstrated to Goethe how a drop of atropine (a toxin from *Atropa belladonna*, or deadly nightshade) led to temporary dilation of the pupil. At one time, the effect made belladonna popular with the ladies — and supposedly the ladies more attractive to men.

Goethe gave Runge a parting gift of a box of coffee beans and told him, "This could be useful for your research." Goethe assumed that coffee contains an anti-

Who Cloned My Cat? Fun Adventures in Biotechnology by R. Renneberg
Copyright © 2011 by Pan Stanford Publishing Pte Ltd
www.panstanford.com
978-981-4267-65-6

dote for atropine — but he was wrong. A year later Runge discovered the "coffee base," the term he would use to describe the stimulant.

Caffeine was, in fact, rediscovered three times: in 1820, also in coffee, by Emmanuel Ferdinand Giese; in 1826 as guaranine in the guarana fruit by Thomas Martius; and in 1827 as theine by Jean-Baptiste Oudry. Christian Jobst proved later in 1838 that caffeine is identical to theine in tea, which is not common knowledge even today.

From 1832 onwards, Runge conducted research in his chemical factory in Schloss Oranienburg, and his work led to further important knowledge. He was the first to isolate quinine, he discovered carbolic acid and aniline in coal tar, and he became a pioneer in the use of natural chemical products and synthetic dyes.

He was also one of the forefathers of paper chromatography, which became the foundation for numerous discoveries in the 20th century. Runge dropped variously colored liquids on blotting papers and identified characteristic structures known as "Runge's pattern figures" (published in 1850 and 1855 in two illustrated books). In his hometown of Oranienburg, Runge was considered a crank and an eccentric. It was only abroad that people appreciated his skills. Isn't that always the way? I am in Hong Kong now!

It's times like these I get a craving for 1,3,7-trimethylxanthine — caffeine I mean! I take mine hot and sweet, thanks.

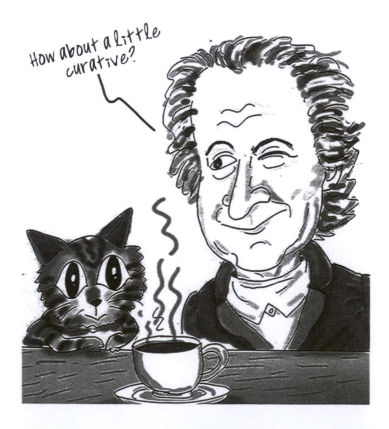

Chapter 48

The Cats and the Bird Flu

Perry the tomcat returned to his Hong Kong home proudly with his prey. But by the very next day, his picture was all over the newspapers: his panicked owner had taken him immediately to the animal shelter — for Perry's prize was a bird and there are grave warnings about bird flu everywhere in China these days. Meanwhile, Ho Choi (Fortune), my tomcat, and my female cat Fortuna are taking a nap beside my laptop. Will I soon be their next victim?

Not too long ago, an entire public swimming pool was emptied out of sheer fear, after a poor bird got inside the building. The *South China Morning Post* reported how 300 people had to quickly leave the pool because the hapless bird had come into contact with the water, and the facility was closed for two hours for cleaning. Later testing found that the bird was negative for the H5N1 virus. The Chinese are an alarmist bunch it seems. But there was similar news in a German newspaper: people were reported to be considering destroying storks' and swallows' nests.

After several cases in Austria, Germany, Thailand and Indonesia, studies are underway to find out if cats can transfer the disease to humans. Eight out of 111 seemingly healthy cats in central Thailand were found to have the antibodies against H5N1, yet were evidently infected. Tigers fed on chicken cadavers have also been infected and have shown early symptoms. According to the World Health Organization though, there is no evidence that cats have passed the virus on to humans.

However, the science journal *Nature* has suggested otherwise. It reported that influenza expert Andrew Jeremijenko discovered a genetically altered H5N1 virus in a healthy kitten in West Java, Indonesia — close to an area infected with bird flu. But this new virus resembled the H5N1 virus found in humans, not in birds! Could the virus have been transferred from humans to cats?

Meanwhile, as Germany's ministers, veterinarians and farmers try to track down suspicious migrating birds, bird-watcher Klemens Steiof from Potsdam and

Who Cloned My Cat? Fun Adventures in Biotechnology by R. Renneberg
Copyright © 2011 by Pan Stanford Publishing Pte Ltd
www.panstanford.com
978-981-4267-65-6

the chief of the Radolfzell Ornithological Station Wolfgang Fiedler continue their discussion about the more likely cause.

Due to space constraints, let's just mention the two most important doubts. Firstly, the 12–15-week delay between the arrival of the migrating birds (potentially carrying the virus) and the first outbreak was too long. Where was the virus during this period? Why wasn't it detected? And secondly, why were there no outbreaks at the birds' most highly frequented destinations and stopovers?

Initial analyses of the genetic connections between different H5N1 strains showed the breeding to have occurred in habitats of Southeast Asia. This suggested that a virus spread by migrating birds was not very likely, but rather it showed a clear connection to the legal and illegal transportation of birds.

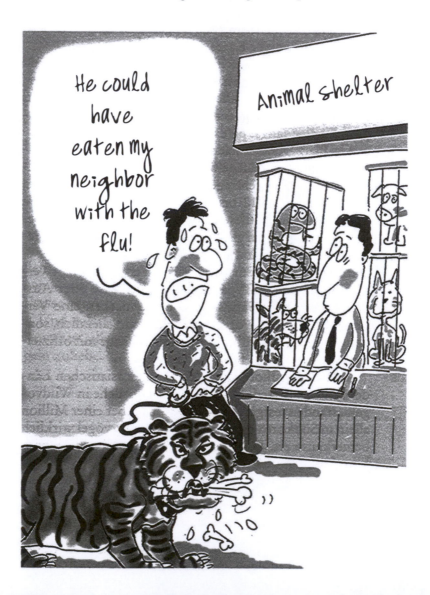

This winter in Japan, South Korea and other Asian countries, there have been no reported virus outbreaks related to migrating birds. This is pretty remarkable considering that there are over a million wintering waterbirds in South Korea alone. Just 500 kilometers away is China, which has been dealing with the disease for the last ten years.

Meanwhile, the feces of over 100,000 healthy migrating birds have been evaluated worldwide, and the highly pathogenic virus was found in only six specimens (in January and March 2005 in eastern China). Moreover, it was quite possible that these six were infected by domestic poultry in the area. These small numbers alone show that the highly pathogenic H5N1 virus has played no significant role for the wild bird population.

Rather than wild birds, it is the global trade in waste and products from the poultry industry that is responsible for spreading the virus; wild birds are not the culprit but the victim. Our current knowledge recognizes that the virus dies with its bird victims on open land. There is no indication that it can survive — without help from farmers. Why are the experiences in Asian countries over the last few decades being so stubbornly ignored?

Wolfgang Fiedler wrote to Klemens Steiof: "I would recommend addressing this subject without ignoring the possibility that wild birds can (also!) carry the virus — just not in the simplistic way that the politicians and the press have treated it."

So, for the time being, my cats Ho Choi and Fortuna are under "house arrest" — but only to keep my university happy. And the birds.

Read more on this subject in Chap. 31, *Hong Kong and the Bird Flu*, p. 67; Chap. 38, *Tamiflu Fever in Hong Kong*, p. 81; Chap. 39, *Save the Wild Birds!* p. 83; and Chap. 65, *From Resignation to WHO*, p. 143.

Chapter 49

Malaria on the Ropes

"Malaria!" My Australian co-worker, Richard Haynes, was bitten by a mosquito in a Malaysian jungle. The insect frantically sucking at a 45-degree angle? The notorious *Anopheles*! But what it didn't know was that Haynes was — and is — the world-renowned chemist who discovered a new anti-malaria medicine. This was one little pathogen that didn't stand a chance.

Malaria is one of the most widespread parasitic diseases in human history. In the world's malarial areas, two billion people are under constant threat. Each year, 200–500 million are infected, and one or two million of them, especially children, die from the disease.

Every year, the malaria that travelers bring back to Europe claims about 12,000 lives. The pathogenic agent responsible for tropical malaria is the one-cell parasite *Plasmodium falciparum*; female *Anopheles* mosquitoes are the carriers. Since the use of the insecticide DDT has been all but outlawed, malaria threatens the world once again.

The first anti-malarial medicine was taken from the *Cinchona* plant species, which produces the alkaloid quinine that nowadays is only used in tonic water to give it its bitter taste. The synthetic drug chloroquine followed in the 1930s, but the parasite started to develop widespread resistance to it in many regions. This is how Haynes, Professor of Organic Chemistry in Hong Kong, came to be asked by pharmaceutical company Bayer to synthesize a new malaria medicine.

Sweet wormwood (*Artemisia annua*), which goes under the name *Qing Hao* in China, has been used in traditional Chinese medicine since ancient times. In the 1980s, it was used to treat malaria. The active ingredient originally used in medicines was artemisinin. Derivatives such as artemether, artesunat and artether are now used in many Asian countries to fight cases of life-threatening, multi-drug-resistant malaria. Yet it does have weaknesses: the substance quickly decomposes in the body and it exhibits neurotoxic features in animal testing.

Who Cloned My Cat? Fun Adventures in Biotechnology by R. Renneberg
Copyright © 2011 by Pan Stanford Publishing Pte Ltd
www.panstanford.com
978-981-4267-65-6

So, the search for a non-toxic derivative is on. Haynes asked himself why the current medicine was neurotoxic. He and his students in Hong Kong painstakingly synthesized hundreds of artemisinin derivatives. Only one showed absolutely no toxic features. It was named artemisone.

Preclinical studies are currently underway at Bayer HealthCare AG in Germany, Austria, England and the US. Compared to the aforementioned artesunat, just one-third of the usual dose of artemisone is required and patients are cured in only two days — quite a sensation! The price of the newly discovered medicine was also an important factor: it had to be a lot less expensive than the old drugs. After all, malaria affects the poorest of the poor, and there is little money to be earned from them.

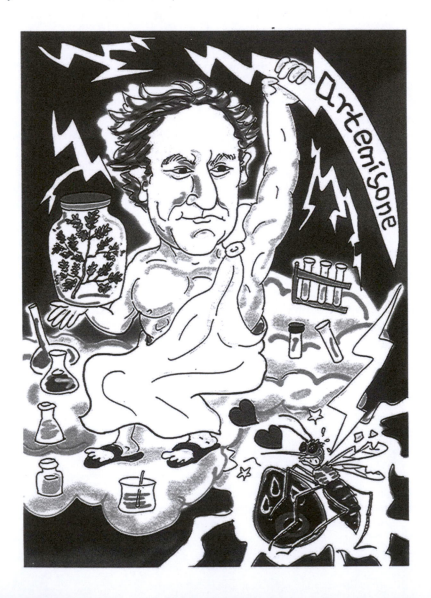

The substance became the feature story in the journal *Angewandte Chemie* in March 2006 — accompanied with a picture of the sweet wormwood plant. The telephone belonging to my now-famous neighbor, Richard, hasn't stopped ringing since. And because Professor Haynes speaks several languages fluently, I can often pick up some Australian-accented German coming from his office: *"Na wunderrrbarrr!"* (How wonderful!) or *"Es klappt herrrvorrragend!"* (It worked superbly!) or *"Danke, aberrr wirrr haben noch viel zu tun!"* (Thank you, but there is still a lot to be done!).

Was that a buzzing sound I just heard? I wonder if a Hong Kong mosquito is about to assume her 45-degree stance and bite me. I probably shouldn't worry, mind you — thanks to the Brits, we're malaria free in Hong Kong.

Chapter 50

Blue Jeans Bacteria Blues

No item of clothing is more authentically American than blue jeans.

The indigo plant (from the Greek *indikon*, meaning Indian) *Indigo tinctoria* and *I. suifructicosa* originate from India and produce a deep blue dye that adheres well to linen and cotton. Initially, in Europe, deep blue garments were reserved for the royals only.

Its popularity really took off thanks to Mister Levi Strauss. The Franconian, who was born in 1829, left for America and arrived in San Francisco in 1853 with a plan to sell tough pants and jackets to gold miners. According to legend, the first pair of Levi's was made of brown tent sheets. Strauss then switched to solid cotton produced in the French city of Nîmes — "de Nîmes," which would become the term used to describe the jeans material: denim.

Indigo blue dye could not be applied directly: the water-insoluble indigo needed to be fermented to water-soluble indigo white first. Fabrics soaked in it then turned blue under the influence of sun and air.

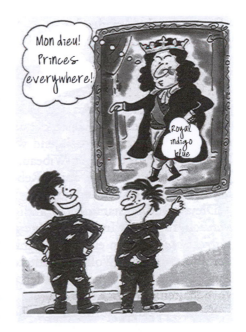

The dyeing industries in Europe started to show an interest in indigo about the same time. The first synthesized dye, mauveine, was discovered serendipitously in 1856 by 18-year-old William Perkin (1836–1907), who was trying to get quinine from coal tar. After that, there was no holding back. In 1880 and 1883, Adolf von Baeyer (1835–1917) successfully synthesized indigo — without knowledge of its chemical

Who Cloned My Cat? Fun Adventures in Biotechnology by R. Renneberg
Copyright © 2011 by Pan Stanford Publishing Pte Ltd
www.panstanford.com
978-981-4267-65-6

structure — and received the 1905 Nobel Prize in Chemistry. BASF, a chemical company from Baden in Germany, attained the patent in 1890, and soon established a dominant position for indigo in the market. The blue jeans revolution had begun.

Indigo dye is about 20 US dollars per kilogram today. Chemically synthesizing it is inexpensive but produces ecologically damaging byproducts: biosynthesis is sorely needed. Genencor International (USA) uses a method whereby coliform bacteria from sugar are used to produce indoxyl from the structurally similar amino acid tryptophan. Indoxyl spontaneously produces indigo in the presence of oxygen. Bacterial indigo cannot be distinguished from the plant-based or industrially produced types, but it is still expensive compared to its purely synthetic cousin.

Jeans are clearly more than just fashion. For one thing, the US textile industry owes it to James Dean and the young rebels of the Sixties for the survival of blue denim.

Chapter 51

Academic Dog-Catching

Chinese people love dogs. And I mean *really*. But two months ago four big stray dogs began to terrorize my university area. They turned up every night, barking loudly and hunting everything in sight. My two cats Fortune and Fortuna and my rabbit Tou-tou have been camping outside my bedroom door shivering with fear. Last week, the dogs knocked over my myna bird's cage, and the poor fellow escaped and hasn't been seen since.

As an owner of a garden in the area, I was chosen to be the academic dog-catcher. I received prompt delivery of a large iron cage equipped with a pressure-sensitive floor. Supposedly, when something ventures in, a mechanism is triggered and the cage door snaps shut. Amazingly, it worked! I caught the culprits!

A note to concerned readers: Eating dog meat has been outlawed in Hong Kong since the time of the pooch-loving Brits, and the city's animal welfare organization, the SPCA — of which I am myself a member — monitors things closely. The captured dogs will be taken to an animal shelter.

Anyway, my being a professor of analytical biotechnology, I got a brilliant idea for a research project right away: developing pressure-sensitive biosensors for dogs.

There already exists a class of pressure-sensitive devices called piezoelectric sensors. They are based around an oscillating quartz crystal whose frequency is correlated with mass. A piezoelectric sensor reacts to anything that binds to its surface. For example: to detect antibodies for a certain virus, a sample of blood is dropped onto the sensor. All sorts of substances will be bound to it and the sensor registers a "false-positive signal."

The same goes for the "dog sensor." The cage was barely opened and my cats were already in for an inspection — followed by my curious rabbit Tou-tou. Separately, each one was too light to produce a signal; this is the sensor's so-called "blind rate." All of them together though set the trap off, thereby producing a false-positive signal.

Who Cloned My Cat? Fun Adventures in Biotechnology by R. Renneberg
Copyright © 2011 by Pan Stanford Publishing Pte Ltd
www.panstanford.com
978-981-4267-65-6

The thing I needed was a bioreceptor — a substance that attracts the analyte specifically (the dogs!) and nothing else. So I popped a juicy roast chicken in the cage. But the next morning it was gone without a trace. The dogs had managed to make off with it without springing the trap.

In the case of biosensors, the bioreceptor has to be *immobilized* (see Chap. 21, *Biochemical Bird Market*, p. 45). In the above example, it is the virus envelope protein that is chemically fixed to the sensor. When a sample of blood is added, only antibodies bind to the virus protein; they fit together perfectly like lock and key. The mass inside the sensor increases and the oscillation slows down: the sought-after antibodies against the virus are detected.

The next night, I put a new chicken in the cage — and *immobilized it* by tying it down firmly. But nothing happened. Maybe it was because there was no Chinese menu hanging in the cage? So, with the help of a Chinese friend, I hung

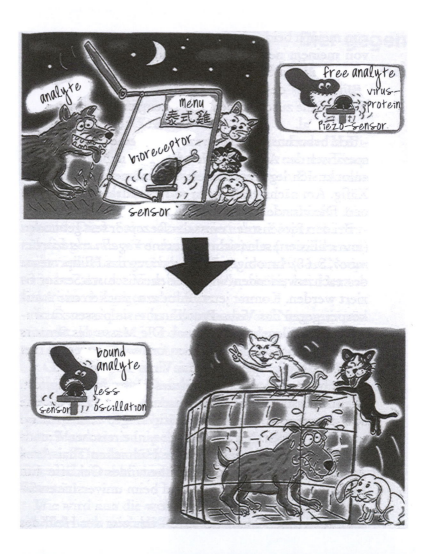

up a sign saying MENU OF THE DAY: THAI CHICKEN — written in Chinese. Very early the following morning there was loud yelping coming from the cage. Sure enough, a large dog had been trapped! My Chinese neighbours, all my colleagues, complained about the noise coming from my garden. A quick call to the university security services and the dog was taken away.

The emails of congratulation came flooding in; I was the hero of the day! And my congratulations to you as well: now you know how piezoelectric biosensors work. Would you have grasped it without my dog example? My poor students have to — in a three-hour lecture!

Chapter 52

Fighting Infection with Beer

It's not only green tea and red wine that are good for your heart and circulation — beer is too! Professor Dietmar Fuchs, together with his team from Innsbruck Medical University in Austria, has demonstrated the infection-inhibiting effects of beer extract.

The Austrian professor is a leading expert in neopterin. This is a substance that alerts our bodies when viral infections occur by being delivered at a high concentration via the blood by immunocompetent cells. It is particularly interesting how neopterin concentration increases markedly during viral infections but only slightly in myocardial infarctions.

In Austria, blood donations are examined for neopterin levels; around two percent will usually be removed because of excessive amounts of the substance. The country has the world's safest donated blood stocks for this reason.

China will likely, as so often of late, put good old Germany to shame by running rapid tests for neopterin on their donated blood in order to make it safer. One can only speculate why this isn't being done in Germany. Reducing blood stocks by two percent is evidently too much for the donation establishments.

Anyway, how were the beneficial effects of beer demonstrated? I volunteered to be a test subject but Prof. Fuchs preferred objective guinea pigs instead: peripheral blood mononuclear cells. These cells are cultivated outside the human body; when artificially inflamed, they generally react the same as when they are inside the body: neopterin is produced and the level of the amino acid tryptophan drops.

The effects of red wine and green tea were studied in Innsbruck a couple of years ago. They were found to influence coronary heart disease favorably and drastically reduce the formation of neopterin.

As for beer: beer extract reduces neopterin levels by about 65 percent whilst raising tryptophan levels. Does that tryptophan boost explain beer's calming effect? Indeed: tryptophan is involved in the synthesis of the "happiness hormone" serotonin. The question is: Which substances in beer are responsible for

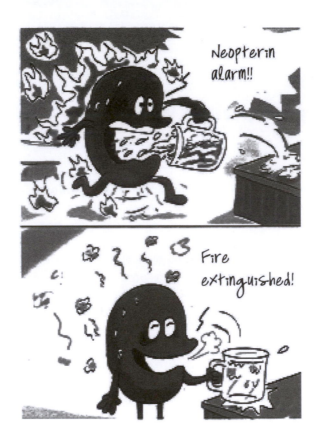

these effects? Probably humulone and isohumulone, the bitter constituents of hops. Fuchs' research is ongoing.

According to Prof. Fuchs, beer can be added to the list of drinks with the potential to inhibit inflammation. But a word of caution: as with wine, the negative effects of consuming alcohol have to be balanced against any positive benefits.

So, go easy when you're quenching your thirst or taming a viral infection!

Chapter 53

The Secret of the Sour Barrels

After Antoni van Leeuwenhoek's discoveries (see Chap. 73, *Leeuwenhoek's Wee Beasties*, p. 161), it took nearly 200 years before microbes grabbed the limelight again. By the middle of the 19th century, large industries had developed throughout Europe, and alcohol was being produced on an industrial scale rather than in small family-run companies.

In 1856 in the French city of Lille, a certain Monsieur Bigo, owner of a distillery, came to see Louis Pasteur, professor of chemistry (for more on Pasteur, see Chap. 55, *Pasteur, Evildoer*, p. 121). Bigo told him about some peculiar changes in his barrels. Instead of turning sugar beet juice into alcohol, they produced some sour-smelling, slimy gray liquid.

Pasteur took his microscope with him and went to the distillery straight away. He took some "healthy" and "unhealthy" samples from the barrels. His microscopic analysis revealed that the "healthy" samples contained small yellow blobs of yeast that clung together like grapes. Much like germinating seeds, shoots were sprouting from the blobs.

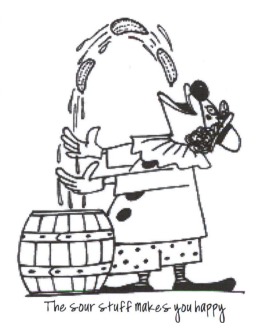

He then investigated the slimy mass and could not find any yeast at all. Instead, he discovered small gray dots, each of which contained a tangle of millions of oscillating rods. The acidic substance these rods seemed to produce turned out to be lactic acid.

As an experiment, Pasteur added a few drops of fluid containing these

The sour stuff makes you happy

Who Cloned My Cat? Fun Adventures in Biotechnology by R. Renneberg
Copyright © 2011 by Pan Stanford Publishing Pte Ltd
www.panstanford.com
978-981-4267-65-6

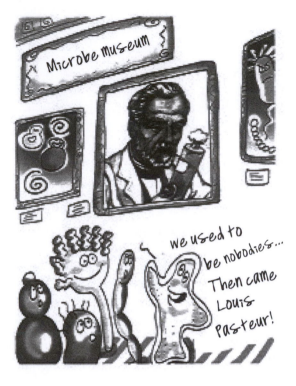

Microbe Museum

we used to be nobodies...
Then came Louis Pasteur!

rods to a flask of clear solution of yeast and sugar. After a short period, all the yeast had disappeared and the rods began to dominate. Again, lactic acid was produced instead of alcohol.

The rods were bacteria — named after the Greek word for rod, *bakterion*. Evidently, the bacteria turned sugar into lactic acid, while the yeast turned sugar into the desired alcohol and carbon dioxide.

Pasteur, who was born in 1822, came from the Jura region of France, and he returned to his hometown regularly on vacation. Not surprisingly, soon after his discovery of lactic acid bacteria, he was asked for advice by the vintners of Arbois. They, too, had trouble with their fermentation. Even the juice of their finest grapes could turn thick, oily and bitter.

Again, Pasteur found tiny bacteria instead of yeast, but this time, they formed chains. More thorough investigations revealed a wide range of bacteria that could spoil wine. Eventually, to the amazement of the vintners, Pasteur was able to predict the taste of a wine sample without even trying it. All he did was look through his microscope and identify the species of yeast or bacteria.

Pasteur also discovered that briefly heating the wine was enough to kill any unwanted bacteria. The same technique was also effective at preventing milk from going sour. This method of killing the majority of microorganisms was named pasteurization, in honor of its inventor.

Even the highest quality raw (unpasteurized) milk contains around 250,000 to 500,000 microbes per milliliter (cubic centimeter)! So, milk is usually briefly heated to 160–165°F (71–74°C), which kills 98 to 99.5% of microorganisms. So-called UHT (ultra-high temperature processed) milk, which keeps for several weeks without refrigeration, has been heated for a short time to a temperature of 248°F (120°C) and is then filled into pasteurized containers.

If microbes had their own museum, Pasteur's portrait would surely be hanging in the main hall.

Chapter 54

The "Red" Crystallographer

GRANDMOTHER WINS NOBEL PRIZE was the headline in an edition of *The Daily Mail* in October 1964. The grandma in question: Dorothy Crowfoot Hodgkin. She was only the third woman to be awarded the Nobel Prize in Chemistry, after Marie Curie and her daughter, Iréne Joliot-Curie.

Dorothy was born in Cairo in 1910 and was the first of four daughters. Her father, John Winter Crowfoot, was a British archeologist and colonial officer. The girls came to England shortly before World War I, and they grew up with their grandmother and a nature-loving nursemaid. Dorothy was allowed to join the chemistry classes at school, which were normally reserved for boys, and she soon set up her own laboratory in the attic of the house where she lived.

She was particularly interested in crystals and in her early years learned about X-ray structural analysis from books. The method allows the determination of crystal structures through their X-ray diffraction patterns. In 1928, she began attending Somerville College in Oxford and was one of the few young women to study chemistry. After obtaining her degree, she continued her studies in Cambridge under the tutelage of John Bernal (1901–1971), who was also an active member of the Communist Party of Great Britain. Whilst there, she established the foundations for X-ray crystallography of important substances such as penicillin and vitamin B12.

When she was 26, she returned to Oxford and became a tutor at her "own" college and got involved in insulin research. She was the first to provide interference pictures of insulin crystals. By 1937, she had received her doctoral degree and married the historian Thomas H. Hodgkin.

In the male-dominated world of science, Crowfoot Hodgkin fought hard for her fellow female colleagues' rights. In 1938, after the birth of her eldest son, she became the first woman to be given maternity leave in Oxford. By the time of her second pregnancy in 1944, all expectant mothers were being given three months' paid maternity leave.

She had two sons and a daughter. After the birth of her first child she began suffering from rheumatoid arthritis. Despite her fingers being crippled by the

Who Cloned My Cat? Fun Adventures in Biotechnology by R. Renneberg
Copyright © 2011 by Pan Stanford Publishing Pte Ltd
www.panstanford.com
978-981-4267-65-6

disease, she still became one of the world's most skilled crystallographers. Eventually, when she was no longer capable of operating the small switches on the X-ray apparatus, she had large levers fitted instead.

By 1946, after four years' work, she had solved the structure of penicillin. Her next challenge was the complex vitamin B_{12} molecule. She presented its structure in 1955, and one year later, she took up a professorship at Oxford. She was awarded the Nobel Prize for her work in 1964, but it was not until 1969 that she published the final structure of insulin — the culmination of 35 years' work.

Aside from her research and teaching activities, Hodgkin was an active and dedicated advocate of world peace. She was president and one of the founders of the Pugwash movement, which seeks to diminish the role of nuclear arms and to promote peace. In 1987 she was awarded the Lenin Peace Prize in Moscow.

Interestingly, the "red" crystallographer once taught a rather conservative 19-year-old chemistry student, Miss Margaret Hilde Roberts — later known as the "Iron Lady" Maggie Thatcher. This reminds me of the education of another top female politician — from Germany. The current German chancellor, Angela Merkel, studied in the former East and spent 12 years at the Central Institute for Physical Chemistry of the Academy of Sciences in Berlin. Unfortunately, she will probably never get a peace prize.

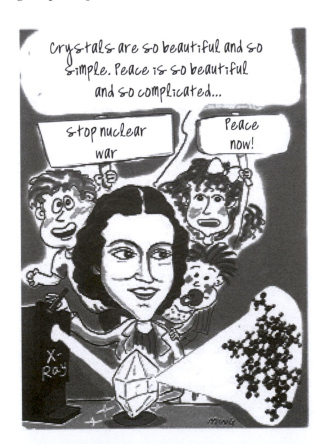

Chapter 55

Pasteur, Evildoer

A case for legal action: A non-medically qualified individual uses material of unknown composition and toxicity to treat patients, including a child, who may be suffering from a potentially fatal illness. The individual does not even try to obtain informed consent, but publishes patients' names and addresses to help publicize some astounding claims. Moreover, like fraudulent quacks the world over, the individual keeps details of the "treatment" secret, so that its validity cannot be independently confirmed. Perhaps worst of all, this reckless person injects his human subjects with an extremely virulent microbe without conducting proper tests on animals beforehand. Some patients die, and a close collaborator who is a medical doctor dissociates himself from his colleague's work. The person who took these risks, yet emerged to thunderous acclaim for his astonishing triumph in defeating rabies, was the great Louis Pasteur.

Pasteur was extremely lucky. As he put it: "Chance favors the prepared mind." Nevertheless, he and other scientists at that time flouted many ethical principles that we practice today.

He postulated that the rabies pathogen would be found in the spinal cord, although it was a completely unknown microbe then. It was made visible under an electron microscope only much later. He also believed that the pathogen could be attenuated by "aging" the spinal cord from rabbits inoculated with spinal cord material from a rabid dog. On July 6, 1885, he injected one Joseph Meister, a young boy badly mauled by a rabid dog, with some of the aged rabbit spinal cord.

The question remains: How can one work in an area where there are few or no certainties at all? How does one come up with the idea of fighting a disease by intentional infection with its pathogen?

It all began with smallpox. By the 11th century, Chinese doctors had already observed that people who had survived a smallpox infection were resistant to recurring infection. In ancient China, toddlers were therefore intentionally infected with smallpox. Given the widespread high infant mortality, the risks associated with this vaccination appeared acceptable.

Who Cloned My Cat? Fun Adventures in Biotechnology **by R. Renneberg**
Copyright © 2011 by Pan Stanford Publishing Pte Ltd
www.panstanford.com
978-981-4267-65-6

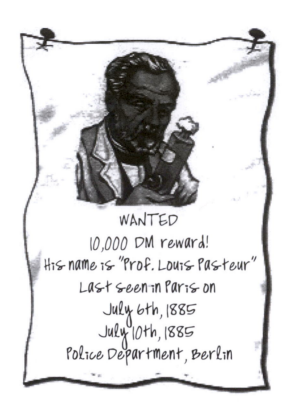

WANTED
10,000 DM reward!
His name is "Prof. Louis Pasteur"
Last seen in Paris on
July 6th, 1885
July 10th, 1885
Police Department, Berlin

The European pioneer who developed a well-tolerated vaccination against smallpox was the British doctor Edward Jenner (1749–1823). He discovered a generally low-risk method with the same purpose in mind by using the innocuous cowpox. However, in his later years, he took a more skeptical approach to the method owing to the resulting side effects — even his own children's health was affected during the experiments.

The true significance of Jenner's discovery, however, was made apparent much later through Louis Pasteur's research. Pasteur had been experimenting on chickens with a pathogen found in cholera-infected birds, *Pasteurella multocida*. One of his cultures had been forgotten in the lab for several weeks before it was used on his chickens. He found that not only did the birds survive the infection but they also became immune to further infections with the pathogen.

Earlier, in 1881, Pasteur had demonstrated in public that sheep could be vaccinated to protect them from anthrax. He was also the savior of silkworm breeding as well as having expounded the scientific principles of wine fermentation. Pasteur was certainly successful — not just lucky.

His triumph against rabies laid the foundation for the establishment of the Pasteur Institute in Paris. Pasteur the "evildoer" was a hero of his time — as he remains today.

Read more on Pasteur's genius in Chap 53, *The Secret of the Sour Barrels*, p. 117.

Chapter 56

The Oil Guzzlers Are Coming

"I won!" cried the usually humble and reserved Indian when he heard the Supreme Court's decision in the case of *Diamond v. Chakrabarty 447 US 303 (1980)*. He had filed a patent in 1971 that had been fighting its way through the courts. His oil-digesting bacterial strain became the first engineered organism in history to be patented in the US, setting a groundbreaking precedent for the biotech industry.

The Indian-born US-based biotechnologist Ananda Mohan Chakrabarty had grown bacteria that could break down the herbicide 2,4,5-T when he was working for General Electric. The herbicide was used in large quantities during the Vietnam War as a component of Agent Orange to defoliate vast areas of jungle.

Afterwards, he went on to grow veritable oil guzzlers. He took plasmids from four *Pseudomonas* strains, each of which degrades octane, camphor, xylene, and naphthalene. These plasmids were then used to create a super-plasmid with the ability to digest all four compounds, which was then reintroduced into the bacteria.

"It's like showing your dog or your cat a couple of new tricks," Chakrabarty told *People* magazine, with typical understatement. The altered bacteria attacked poisonous crude oil residues with a vengeance and they were intended to be used to quickly clean up large oil slicks, such as those created in oil tanker disasters. The massive numbers of microorganisms would later be devoured by organisms higher up in the food chain.

However, Chakrabarty's oil guzzlers have never been used. Restrictions on the release of genetically modified bacteria into the environment have seen to that.

When the oil tanker *Exxon Valdez* was stranded on the Alaskan coast in 1989, and an estimated 250,000 seabirds were killed, conventionally bred bacteria were used. While most of the 38,000 tons of spilled oil were pumped off and filtered, the coating of oil on rocks and pebbles was broken down by natural microbes. Their growth was enhanced by the addition of phosphate and nitrate "fertilizers."

In fact, millions of tons of crude end up in the seas every year, but spectacular oil tanker disasters like that of the *Exxon Valdez* are only responsible for a small

Who Cloned My Cat? Fun Adventures in Biotechnology by R. Renneberg
Copyright © 2011 by Pan Stanford Publishing Pte Ltd
www.panstanford.com
978-981-4267-65-6

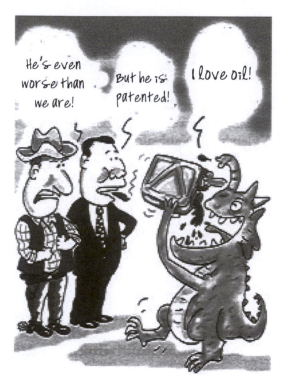

percentage of overall oil pollution. The illegal cleaning of empty tankers in the open sea as well as the dumping of effluent into rivers are the key sources of the pollution.

Cleaning up petroleum-contaminated soil (under gas stations, for example) is more complicated. After German reunification, soil remediation became a major issue in the former East Germany. Seven-foot-high heaps of soil were inoculated with special microbes, aerated and stirred. In most cases, after two weeks, more than 90 percent of the pollutants were broken down. Several companies soon began earning a fortune.

German writer and biologist Bernhard Kegel has imagined the oil guzzlers in a rather different light. In his readable thriller "Sexy Sons," Kegel describes a frightening scenario: not only does the cloning of the boss of a global environmental protection company go horribly wrong, but genetically engineered, oil-digesting super-microbes are maliciously introduced into oil wells — with disastrous consequences!

So what would happen if the oil guzzlers really reached the oil fields? Who knows? But there would then surely no longer be any justification for military intervention in the Middle East.

Remark: In 2010, the US faced the biggest oil spill in human history after a BP-managed offshore drilling platform exploded and sank.

Chapter 57

Antibiotic Stinky White Fungus

What did Pasteur say again? Chance favors the prepared mind? Well, take the microbiologist Gary Strobel, who lives in Montana, a US state containing Earth's northernmost rainforest. He has a passion for research into endophytes, microorganisms that use plants as hosts.

On his treks, he takes samples from various plants, and in 1993, he found a fungus on the bark of a Pacific yew in Northwest Montana. Strobel was convinced that microbes on plants produce similar products to their hosts. The fungus he isolated was named *Taxomyces andreanae* after the host yew (*Taxus*) and — according to gentlemanly custom — the lady on the team, Andrea.

After culturing the fungus and analyzing the products, Strobel still had not found what he was looking for, but he continued to study the structure over and over. Eventually, his persistence paid off: the little fungus finally yielded taxol — a substance that had been shown to exhibit anti-cancer activity in humans.

In 1997 the US Patent Office granted patents for various fungi that produced taxol. Further tests showed that *Taxomyces andreanae* had many relatives and these other species of the same genus were part of a greater breakthrough. One of the fungus families from the Asian yew produces a thousand times the amount of taxol.

Taxol is one of the most promising anti-tumor drugs of the last three decades. In 2008, Brian Drucker from Oregon got the Lasker Award — often called "the small Nobel Prize" — for his work on Taxol. It is essential that Taxol can be produced at low cost and in large quantities. The worldwide market was worth one billion US dollars in 2000. Today, it stands at about two billion US dollars for all taxol varieties. Sadly, although it has dramatically prolonged the survival time of patients, it is not a cure for cancer. Many patients develop a resistance to the drug and many tumors just do not respond to it. So, the search for possible modifications goes on.

Unfortunately, Strobel's fungus produced taxol in quantities that were too tiny to be competitive. Nevertheless, he had still made the brilliant fundamental discovery that microbial parasites imitate their host's chemistry and manufacture the same chemical compounds. If the microbe could be isolated and cultured, it might

Who Cloned My Cat? Fun Adventures in Biotechnology by R. Renneberg
Copyright © 2011 by Pan Stanford Publishing Pte Ltd
www.panstanford.com
978-981-4267-65-6

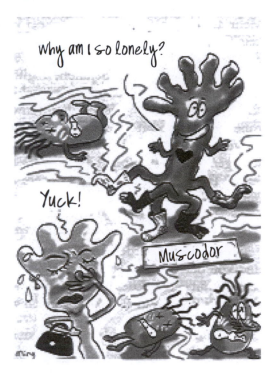

be a discovery of equivalent magnitude to penicillin — and there are thousands of other fungi! Here's the problem: if the hosts continue to be systematically destroyed — as is happening in the rainforests right now — then these valuable microbes will be gone as well.

Gary Strobel retired at the age of 67, but he never stopped his research. He has traveled to rainforests all over the world for 20 years, collecting bark and twigs and cultivating their "inhabitants."

In 1999, he came upon another unusual phenomenon: during the transportation of his fungus samples, all of the those in the open containers arrived safely but only one of those in his closed containers survived.

Strobel was perplexed. But then came the eureka moment: the surviving endophytic fungus had evidently produced gases (volatile organic compounds, VOCs) that had killed the other fungi! He named the fungus *Muscodor albus* — stinky white fungus. Although Strobel found more than 30 different substances in the VOCs, no individual compound was found to be lethal to animals or plants. In combination, though harmless to us, they were found to kill many pathogens that affect both plants and humans.

Recognizing its potential, Strobel patented his microscopic stinky white fungus. Now the clients are lining up. One company wants to use *Muscodor* to remove microbes that spoil fruit during transportation and storage. Another wants to make use of them in portable toilets. The fungus can be dried and shrink-wrapped and then subsequently revived when moistened. The gases it produces can then neutralize other odors and kill pathogenic bacteria.

Such toilets have been used in national parks — as well as by the US Army. One wonders whether these odor-free *Muscodor* toilets might do something for the popularity of American GIs around the world!

Chapter 58

Praising Ginger

Oh no! Not seasickness too?! I felt pretty queasy on the ship from Cape Town to Robben Island. The cutter that may have carried Nelson Mandela and his comrades to prison was lurching heavily. Luckily for me though, my girlfriend Louiza had some "ginger sticks" in my backpack!

Ginger is one secret Chinese remedy that has been overlooked in Germany. Not so in England and the US, where ginger ale, ginger lemonade, ginger sweets and even ginger ice cream are all very popular.

The ginger plant (*Zingiber officinale*) has no major root but rather its characteristic rootstocks (rhizomes). It can be eaten raw or cooked — though fresh and uncooked, it has a distinctly pungent taste. Ginger has a mild aroma and its distinctive flavor comes from the compounds gingerol and zingerone. It is mainly made up of about three percent essential oil and an additional 30 famous phytochemicals.

For 3000 years, ginger has been used everywhere in China — but mostly in the kitchen. It has been made into an alcoholic liqueur in Canton since the Qing Dynasty (the gentleman in the top-left of the cartoon is making a toast); it is a component of cough sweets; and it has been used to ease seasickness.

For the Chinese, ginger is a "heaty" *yang* substance and is used for all kinds of physical ailments. So, it's no surprise that the biomedical field has long taken an interest in understanding the compounds contained in this talented root. It is indeed astonishing just how many benefits have been linked to this single plant: reducing inflammation, thrombosis prevention, controlling blood pressure, regulating kidney function, and much more.

The effects of the ingredients in ginger are often compared with aspirin. And this is not something plucked out of thin air. Ginger contains the inhibitor cyclooxygenase (COX), a prostaglandin synthesis enzyme that plays an important role in inflammation and blood clotting (see Chap. 22, *One Pill for (Almost) Everything?* p. 47 and Chap. 41, *Mussel Extract Takes On Vioxx®*, p. 87). Gingerol

Who Cloned My Cat? Fun Adventures in Biotechnology by R. Renneberg
Copyright © 2011 by Pan Stanford Publishing Pte Ltd
www.panstanford.com
978-981-4267-65-6

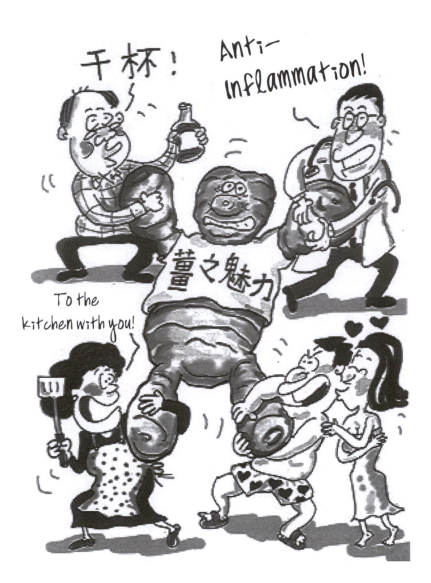

also resembles aspirin in structure and it reduces the risk of blood vessel blockage and arteriosclerosis — with no known side effects.

Ginger helps sufferers of headaches and migraines, too. Against allergies, rheumatism, blood circulation diseases, and even some types cancer (owing to the aforementioned cyclooxygenase), it has also been shown to have healing effects. But a great deal of research is still needed to explain the connections.

In addition, it has been assumed that ginger has antibacterial effects that work against the ulcer-causing *Helicobacter* in the stomach. Slices of ginger are often added to fish dishes in Hong Kong to keep them fresh and to temper the smell.

However, like everything else in life, it is best not to overdo it. People taking the anticoagulant warfarin are warned against taking ginger, as are those who have gallstones because ginger stimulates bile acid production. Moreover, ginger is not well tolerated by everyone. I, for one, have too much "heaty" *yang* (according to the Chinese), so I shouldn't be adding fuel to the fire.

Lesser-known powers are hiding in the ginger bulb as well — like helping you with your hangover. A little nibble before (or during) enjoying a tipple will (hopefully) mean you'll wake up the next morning without that splitting headache (see Chap. 6, *Hanging on to Hangovers*, p. 11).

How about making ginger available as pills? The latest research from Baltimore (USA), surprisingly, could not show a connection between death rates caused by heart and circulatory diseases and the consumption of vitamin C, E and β-carotene tablets. In contrast, fruits and vegetables, which contain lots of vitamin C, E and β-carotene, have shown positive results. It seems that a well-balanced diet is enough to keep one healthy; there's really no need for extra vitamins or food supplements. The same goes for ginger pills.

When it comes to getting seasick, though, my ginger sticks saved me. If you ask me, ginger belongs in every intrepid traveler's baggage. Talking about dream trips, I've just read that besides its calming effects on the stomach, ginger is also an effective aphrodisiac (see the cartoon on the two covers in the lower-right corner)…

Chapter 59

Litmus and Hemp

"The litmus test, ladies and gentlemen, is, um, in this case… err… blah, blah, blah…" How many times have we heard this? The litmus test is surely the only chemical test that has made its way into popular culture — and especially the vocabulary of political speechwriters. But who knows what this test really is? I asked my Chinese chemist colleagues about the "litmus formula" and they all shook their heads. One of them at least managed: "A complex mix that works."

The name "litmus" as well as the product itself originates from the Netherlands. There, in the 16th century, the lichens *Ochrolechia* and *Lecanora* were collected, ground up and mixed with urine, lime and potassium carbonate. During several weeks of fermentation, the color of the mixture would turn slowly from red to purple and then to blue. The precious blue pigment could then be extracted, and it was used mainly to dye the wool and silk robes of the royals. The rich, deep colors were not very lasting, however.

Maybe, once upon a time, at a royal dinner with his future queen, a prince spilled some vinegar on her deep blue robe and suddenly it had red spots all over it. The royal physician would, of course, have been fascinated by this spectacle, and a bright idea was soon on its way…

In fact, Robert Boyle (1627–1691), one of the fathers of modern chemistry — who defined the term "analysis" — was the first person to carry out the litmus test. It was in 1660 that he determined the acidity measures of solutions that we all know today as pH values.

The determination of acidity using litmus paper is quite simple: the paper turns red if the solution is acidic, and blue if it is alkaline. Robert Boyle seems to have used material extracted from lichens. However, the French also claim the invention of litmus paper as their own. French star chemist Louis Gay-Lussac (1778–1850) is said to have developed litmus paper at the beginning of the 19th century in Paris.

The paper for the litmus test was first plunged into boiling litmus broth, and then dried and placed in special vessels that prevent light from entering. Today, the best litmus producers are the lichens *Roccella tinctoria* from the Mediterranean Sea and *Ochrolechia tartarea* from the Netherlands.

Who Cloned My Cat? Fun Adventures in Biotechnology by R. Renneberg
Copyright © 2011 by Pan Stanford Publishing Pte Ltd
www.panstanford.com
978-981-4267-65-6

There are about 15,000 kinds of lichens. They are the result of a symbiosis between living algae and fungus. The algae take care of photosynthesis, and the fungus depends on them and grows on the organic substrate. The result is the production of a raft of substances, including lichen acids, and they have antibacterial effects that keep other fungi at bay. Even though lichens actually consist of two living organisms, they go under one name. Lichens can be found everywhere — on bark, stones and walls. They are also environmentally sensitive indicators since poor air quality in cities prevents them from thriving.

Netherlanders are still the biggest producers of litmus tests and pH meters. When I asked a practically minded colleague in Groningen why this is the case, he grinned, pointed at some pots of beautiful plants — which I was not familiar with — and said, "They're completely legal! Hemp only grows at certain pH values. If the soil is too acidic, the hemp plant will not produce any female blossoms. Then there will be no big flowers — and nothing to smoke or laugh about." He left me speechless in his office. Time for a *legal* Dutch smoking break, I guess.

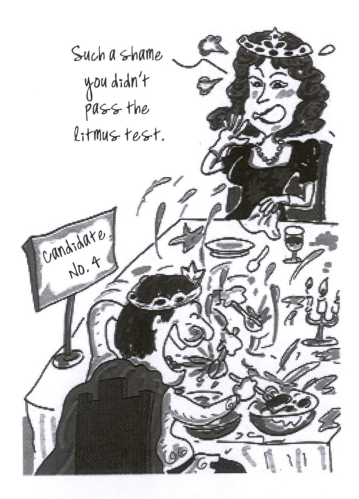

Chapter 60

Another Spoonful of Red Wine?

Georges Halpern is 71 years old and looks much younger than me (according to him anyway). A colleague and a pharmacy professor at the Hong Kong Polytechnic University, he is also a nutritionist. As a young French Jew, he was forced to hide from the Nazis in the woods for an entire year, and during that difficult time, he stayed alive by eating anything edible that he could find.

Whenever we meet, red wine shows up on the table. After finishing the first bottle, I always try to find out the secret of his youthful good looks.

Let's take the wine for starters. Is there anything new to say about it? Wine contains 8 to 14 percent alcohol by volume. The effect of alcohol on mortality in the industrialized world follows a J-shaped curve. Compared to nondrinkers, those who drink moderately live longer. But among those who drink to excess, the death rate increases sharply.

The healthy components of wine are antioxidants from grapes called polyphenols. Red wine contains 900 to 2,500 milligrams of polyphenols per liter; white wine only has 190 to 290 milligrams. One glass of red wine (150 milliliters) provides as much antioxidant as there is in 12 glasses of white wine, two cups of tea, five apples, 100 grams of onions, half a liter of beer, seven glasses of orange juice, or 20 glasses of apple juice.

The Copenhagen City Mortality Study has concluded that wine drinkers have a significantly lower mortality than nondrinkers. Hundreds of studies have confirmed that moderate red wine consumption protects against circulatory diseases. The most important mechanism is the protection from oxidization of the "bad" lipoproteins (LDLs). Oxidized LDLs can actively embed themselves into vessel walls and cause inflammation. On the other hand, "good" HDLs, which transport lipids away, are activated by wine phenols.

After finishing his first glass, Georges orders some food. "Most importantly, in order to make use of all the benefits of a good red wine, it must be accompanied by a good dinner," he points out. Indeed, a study over a seven-year period of 8,647 men and 6,521 women between the ages of 30 and 59 has shown how those drinking

Who Cloned My Cat? Fun Adventures in Biotechnology by R. Renneberg
Copyright © 2011 by Pan Stanford Publishing Pte Ltd
www.panstanford.com
978-981-4267-65-6

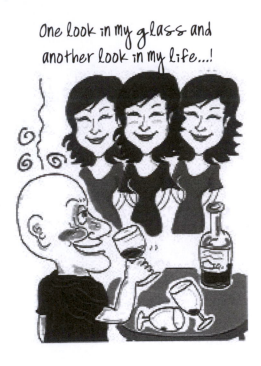

One look in my glass and another look in my life...!

without food died earlier than those who enjoyed their wine with a meal.

Georges does a simple calculation: if every American had two glasses of red wine with their meals every day, heart and circulatory diseases (accounting for half of all deaths) would reduce by 40 percent. Plus, it would save 40 billion US dollars per year! (Hope the Minister of Health reads this!)

The Romans conquered half of the world — without getting diarrhea. The secret was red wine in their drinking water: the polyphenols effectively killed off bacteria, salmonella and *Escherichia coli*. Moderate amounts of wine (or green tea) can also kill *Helicobacter pylori*, a bacterium responsible for gastric ulcers.

According to the Copenhagen Study, examining 3,777 people over 65 years old, red wine protects against stroke and even improves memory. 318 of them drank 250–500 milliliters of red wine daily and they passed the memory tests with flying colors.

One last question remains: if it's so easy, why don't all wine drinkers look as youthful and fresh-faced as the 71-year-old professor?

"Well, when you're enjoying your red wine, you also have to look deeply into the eyes of a gorgeous woman," says Georges, clinking glasses with his beautiful, young Chinese assistant.

Chapter 61

DNA Caps

At first glance, the end portions of chromosomes are quite boring. The order of the bases in this region is repeated hundreds of times in short, characteristic patterns: GGGGTT GGGGTT GGGGTT, etc. So why is it important for cells that these ends are as long as possible?

The mystery now seems to have been solved, and the discoverers received the 2006 Lasker Award for Basic Medicine along with 100,000 US dollars in prize money. The Lasker Award is often considered a precursor to the Nobel Prize. The honorees are Elizabeth Blackburn (University of California, San Francisco), Carol Greider (Johns Hopkins University) and Jack Szostak (Harvard Medical School).

During division of a healthy cell, a part of the DNA strand is always lost. The end portion of a chromosome, called a telomere (from the Greek: *telos* for "end" and *meros* for "part"), gets shorter and shorter with each division until the cell eventually dies. The function of the telomere "caps" at the end of each chromosome is to prevent the loss of genetic information.

The aglets or sheaths at the ends of shoelaces provide a rough analogy: if an aglet is lost, the shoelace unravels. In the human body, these chromosome-protecting caps start with lengths of up to 20,000 base pairs. This limits the number of cell divisions in the body to 50 to 60 times.

Lisa Blackburn discovered the telomere in the single-cell *Tetrahymena* as a postdoctoral student at Yale University. In 1980, while working at a laboratory in the University of California, Berkeley, she met the yeast geneticist Jack Szostak at a conference. Shortly after, she placed the repetitive *Tetrahymena* sequences in budding yeast cells. But the expected destruction did not take place: the single-cell DNA was protected by the telomere!

After further experiments, Blackburn and Szostak postulated that an enzyme must be attaching the telomere to the DNA. It was Carol Greiner, a student at Blackburn's laboratory, who discovered the enzyme telomerase and showed how it functioned. In its active nucleus, the telomerase has ribonucleic acid (RNA) "teeth": one part of the RNA sequence is CCCCAA, which is the exact

Who Cloned My Cat? Fun Adventures in Biotechnology **by R. Renneberg**
Copyright © 2011 by Pan Stanford Publishing Pte Ltd
www.panstanford.com
978-981-4267-65-6

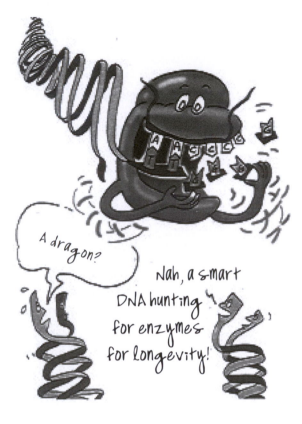

complement to GGGGTT in the telomere DNA.

Using yeast cells, Szostak showed how chromosomes without telomerase become shorter after each division; essentially, cells age.

But can't this be stopped? Wouldn't that reveal the secret of eternal youth or even immortality? Or at the very least allow us to maintain our cells in their best condition?

In 1998, it was discovered that — in tissue cultures at least — the lifespan of human cells could be extended if telomerase could be built in. Still, the principle only applies to cells that undergo frequent division, such as those from bone marrow, skin or hair. Fortunately, it is just these kinds of cells that are needed for therapeutic purposes.

What about cancer cells? They seem to have "super" telomerase. If things work as described above, then a telomerase inhibitor could be a great way of fighting cancer — even in advanced stages.

As with the rest of life, there are always two sides — even when it comes to the cell. Perhaps immortality has too high a price… I would rather follow the advice of the hedonist writer Peter Ustinov: "Children are the only form of immortality that we can be sure of."

Read more on this subject in Reinhard Renneberg's *Biotechnology for Beginners*, Academic Press, New York, 2008.

Chapter 62

Take the Old One

In 1996, Dolly became the first mammal to be cloned via somatic cell nuclear transfer (SCNT). More than a dozen species of mammals have since been cloned using this technology (see Chap. 26, *Just as Long as It Catches Mice!* p. 55; Chap. 33, *Going to the Dogs?* p. 71 and Chap. 44, *Snuppy, Made in Korea*, p. 93).

Success rates of between one and five percent don't sound like much, but if embryonic stem cells (ES cells) are used as donors instead of somatic cells, the rate is a factor of five to ten higher.

Stem cells are body cells that are not yet differentiated. They are not yet specialized as, for example, skin or liver cells. A mechanism — which is not yet fully understood — creates two kinds of daughter cells: organ-specific cells and new stem cells. The decision is mainly made under the influence of the cell's surroundings.

The use of ES cells was quickly labeled "baby homicides" by some. This was not without good reason: it was feared that embryos would be cultured to provide spare parts for (rich) patients and killed at the blastocyst stage.

So stem-cell and clone scientists frantically began looking for politically correct alternatives — and they discovered adult stem cells. Patients suffering myocardial infarctions, leukemia and other chronic diseases were soon being treated using this method, and the treatments were successful to some extent. The adult stem cells were taken from bone marrow or umbilical cord blood. Embryonic stem-cell research remains a long way off in the context of such successes — and cloning is an even more remote possibility. Maybe the whole ES-cell hysteria was unnecessary?

It now seems like stem cells are rather dispensable. Professor Tao Cheng and his team from Pittsburgh University in Pennsylvania have managed to clone mice from completely differentiated body cells! Cheng has had an interesting career, starting as a Chinese army doctor before becoming a professor in the US. At the same time, he is a professor at the Second Military Medical University in Shanghai, and surely as an officer of the People's Liberation Army as well.

Who Cloned My Cat? Fun Adventures in Biotechnology by R. Renneberg
Copyright © 2011 by Pan Stanford Publishing Pte Ltd
www.panstanford.com
978-981-4267-65-6

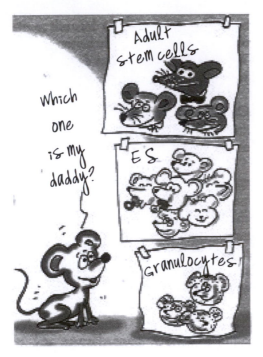

In their SCNT work, Cheng's co-workers Li Ying Sung and Shaorong Gao took hematopoietic cells at various differentiation stages: adult stem cells, progenitor cells and granulocytes. The cell nuclei were injected into fertilized egg cells in different stages of development. They developed from the blastocyst stage to embryos. Surprisingly, the nuclei from old, mature cells were the best — unlike the adult stem cells, which proved disappointing.

Next, the mouse embryos were transplanted into their surrogate mothers. Of 1,300 nuclear transfers of granulocytes, 35 percent reached the blastocyst stage and just two clones survived. The team declared that for the first time cloning from completely differentiated body cells had been successful. Critics remarked that high blastocyst efficiency had only recently been demonstrated. Others were thrilled. Let's wait and see how things turn out.

Old truths do not last long in science — but it seems old cells are making headway.

An old couplet by Berlin chansonnier Otto Reutter would be fitting here:

Nehm'n Se'n Alten, nehm'n Se'n Alten!
Der ist froh, wenn Sie'n behalten.
Der bleibt treu in Ewigkeit, wird immer treuer mit der Zeit.
Nehm'n Se'n Alten, nehm'n Se'n Alten!

Take an old one, take an old one!
He'll be happy if you keep him.
He'll be faithful forever and even more with time.
Take an old one, take an old one!

Chapter 63

Was Mozart's Starling a Composer?

Wolfgang Amadeus Mozart (1756–1791) in a graveyard. After a ceremonial hymn and a self-recited poem, he buried his friend — a starling. According to his records, Mozart bought the bird on May 27, 1784. The starling could whistle the tune from his Piano Concerto No. 3 in G major. While Mozart composed on his piano, the starling sang along cheerfully in modulation. "It was so beautiful!" he wrote on a sheet of music, adopting the starling's version for the last movement. "A Musical Joke" (Köchel catalogue no. 522) is believed to have been inspired by the starling as well.

Starlings can even sing in harmony, says Luis Baptista, an ornithologist at the California Academy of Sciences. Females learn from their mothers and males learn from their fathers. Some can even sing, as in classical music, in sonata form with exposition, development, recapitulation and coda.

Fernando Nottebohm from Rockefeller University is a bird lover — which makes him instantly likeable in my eyes. In 1976, he was the first to verify anatomically the musical center of a songbird's brain. Gender plays an important role: the region of the brain used for singing in the male zebra finch is anatomically five times bigger than in the female. This makes sense because the male sings to advertise himself while the female sits quietly on her eggs in order not to give away the location of her nest to predators. Accordingly, the singing center of male canaries' brains shrinks outside the breeding season.

Nottebohm discovered another surprise from birds in 1984: new neural cells can be created in adult brains. Birds require new neurons to store new experiences; their brains are so small that their recording capacity is limited. When canaries reach the end of the breeding season, the part of their brains used for singing will shrink. But new melodies are needed by the next breeding season, so new neural cells will be created. While this process takes place rather abruptly in canaries, the zebra finch brain produces new neurons continuously.

Nottebohm also analyzed the influence of communication partners on neuron formation among adult zebra finches. He divided them into three

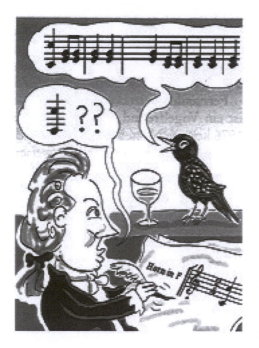

groups: singles, pairs, and a mixed group of about 45 birds.

After 40 days, the brain area used for singing was studied, and it was found that the birds in the large group formed about 30 percent more new neurons than singles and pairs. Singing males in the big group had twice as many new neurons compared with singing males in the singles and the pairs group.

Nottebohm assumed that the finches try to identify each member by its characteristic singing pattern: the bigger the group, the more storage is needed in their brains.

Although it had long been known that social animals have better memories than individualistic ones, there had been no definitive evidence that the number of animals in a group is an important factor as well. The only question now is: Can the results from finch studies also be applied to humans? Yes — at least theoretically, say neurobiologists.

Committed loners and couch potatoes who immediately want to plunge into the world of communication in order to revive their neurons should probably start small — by hanging out with zebra finches!

Chapter 64

Much Smoke About the Heart

The capital of China on an autumn day: sunny but cold. All around the city were photographs of elephants and zebras, and an African hand shaking a Chinese hand: Beijing's China-Africa summit was in full swing. At the same time, ten thousand Chinese cardiologists and nurses were gathered at the 14th Great Wall International Congress of Cardiology. Inside the giant congress halls, giant hearts were pulsating on giant screens. I had travelled to the congress from Hong Kong to show off our "CardioDetect" — the world's fastest heart infarction test — which was developed in Berlin-Buch and Hong Kong and now produced at low cost in China.

One is spoilt for choice when there are eight presentations running concurrently. I went to a talk by one of the stars of the West, "inflammation guru" Peter Libby, presently chief of cardiovascular medicine at Brigham and Women's Hospital in Boston and a professor at Harvard University. There wasn't much that was new to me in Libby's presentation (most of the content of his speech can be found in an issue of *Scientific American* from July 2002), but the Chinese attendees were enthralled by his easy charm.

Perhaps this was hardly surprising as in a nearby auditorium a Chinese speaker, talking on the subject of "Smoking and the Heart," was sending the attending doctors to sleep. The speaker looked and spoke like a chain smoker, and even had a rather suspicious cough. Incidentally, there are an estimated 350 million smokers in China.

Meanwhile, Libby, the American entertainer, was in good form. A couple of years ago, most doctors would explain arteriosclerosis to their patients by comparing it to the calcification in water pipes. Fatty materials build up slowly on arterial walls and the blood vessels are gradually clogged with calcium. But this was all wrong: arterial walls are not stiff and passive like pipes. They are made of living cells, which are crucial in the forming and development of arteriosclerotic deposits. Moreover, the plaque deposition does not take place on the arterial walls but within them.

Who Cloned My Cat? Fun Adventures in Biotechnology by R. Renneberg
Copyright © 2011 by Pan Stanford Publishing Pte Ltd
www.panstanford.com
978-981-4267-65-6

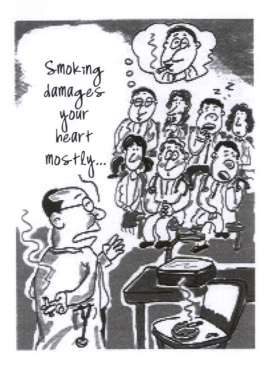

According to the latest thinking, inflammation triggers arteriosclerosis and causes fat deposition in arterial walls. It can also cause vessel walls to suddenly rip open. The risk of blood clotting and arterial blockage then becomes particularly high. This results in the most frightening consequence of arteriosclerosis: heart infarction or stroke.

Too much "bad" cholesterol (LDL) is one of the triggers of inflammation reactions in the arteries.

In order to identify patients most at risk, Libby suggests measuring inflammation levels in addition to the well-established blood test for cholesterol. A combination of lipid level and C-reactive protein (CRP) measurements is ideal, according to Libby. Some of his colleagues from the West have their doubts about this — but they were not there in Beijing.

What about the roles other risk factors play in inflammation reactions? Diabetes increases glucose levels in blood, causing the "sweetening" of protein and intensifying LDL-induced inflammation. Healthy nutrition, regular physical activity and, if necessary, weight reduction can lower the risk of heart attacks and adult-onset diabetes. Smoking, on the other hand, helps the formation of strongly reactive oxidants and with it the oxidation of LDL components.

When Libby left the auditorium after long applause and I went to greet him, we found ourselves gasping for air in front of an impenetrable Great Wall of Chinese cigarette smoke. The neighboring room had finished five minutes earlier.

Read more on this subject in Chap. 15, *Helping Hands for Your Heart*, p. 31.

Chapter 65

From Resignation to WHO

At the latest Beijing China-Africa summit, which involved some 48 African countries, Hu Jintao, President of the People's Republic of China, heralded Margaret Chan, Hong Kong bird flu expert, as a candidate for chief of the World Health Organization (WHO). Hu expressed his humble hope that African countries would support her. Her appointment was indeed to be.

Chan's experience as Hong Kong's Health Minister during the 1997 bird flu and the deadly lung disease SARS outbreaks in 2003 were highly praised before the election. But how do the people of her home country view her experience?

Ming Pao, one of Hong Kong's biggest newspapers, wrote that because of Chan's failures and lack of resolve, around 300 died of SARS; her election was a disgrace for the WHO.

"She does not have the expertise to deal with international health issues. She hesitated far too long before analyzing the spread of SARS in Hong Kong to undertake effective action later; thus, more people were infected," said one story. A banner during one demonstration read: MARGARET CHAN HAS NO CONSCIENCE. Some believe that Chan followed Beijing's orders and covered up the real scale of the SARS problem.

It was not until the courageous actions of a Chinese doctor named Jiang Yanyong that the world learned the truth. The virus would eventually spread from Hong Kong to the rest of the world and claim 800 human lives worldwide. Heavy criticism from the public forced her to resign in August 2003. In 2004, the Hong Kong legislature unanimously concluded that Chan had reacted too slowly and missed the opportunity to combat the epidemic.

The Health Ministry in China took a very different stance, saying that Chan had dealt with the SARS issue in Hong Kong "with respect for collective interests." They lauded the expertise of their "Hong Kong virus expert" at an international conference on health in Macao and endorsed her candidacy for the position of WHO chief.

In 1997, when the first case of bird flu was made known to the public, she told Hong Kongers that it was still safe to eat chicken. Shortly after, the city suffered a

Who Cloned My Cat? Fun Adventures in Biotechnology by R. Renneberg
Copyright © 2011 by Pan Stanford Publishing Pte Ltd
www.panstanford.com
978-981-4267-65-6

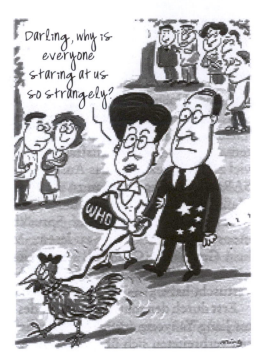

Darling, why is everyone staring at us so strangely?

massive outbreak. There were 18 infected patients and five of them died. However, Chan made what was, in my opinion, a courageous decision: 1.4 million chickens, ducks and geese were slaughtered within a couple of days to prevent further spread of the virus.

What made the WHO pick Chan anyway? They might hope that, with Chan on top, Beijing will be seen to be reporting outbreaks efficiently and making crucial information available at the proper time. Shortly before Chan's election, the Chinese Ministry of Agriculture hadn't submitted a single bird flu virus sample since 2004. Directly after, the WHO confirmed that 20 samples had been sent to their laboratory in the US.

This change of heart seems rather too sudden. Is it sincere? My Chinese friends calm me down: "We are 100 percent sure about that! China will be putting on an amazing show for the Beijing Olympics in 2008 — and nothing will get in the way of the greatest Olympics of all time. So the bird flu virus is now public enemy number one!"

Read more about bird flu in Chap. 31, *Hong Kong and the Bird Flu*, p. 67; Chap. 39, *Save the Wild Birds!* p. 83 and Chap. 48, *The Cats and the Bird Flu*, p. 101.

Chapter 66

"West Gelman" Eggs for Sale!

Consumers of fish in Hong Kong got a rude shock one day: Malachite Green was found in freshwater fish imported from mainland China. Used to disinfect water, Malachite Green (triphenylcarbenium chloride) is an effective treatment against parasites and fungal infections in fish and fish eggs. It's cheap and it's easy to get.

However, fish contaminated with Malachite Green have been shown to be harmful to human health. Suspected of being responsible for tumor formation, this triphenylmethanol dye has been outlawed in Europe for use in fish food for some time now. Imported fish are not allowed to come into contact with the substance either.

Chinese fish farmers are facing a dilemma. Overfishing has increased greatly due to the rapid growth in fish consumption, and the quantities of fish caught in the world's oceans are dropping. The result has been a rise in the number of fish farms, but intensive husbandry has led to parasite affliction, and farmers have been forced by greed, or even just despair, to use illegal chemicals. Imports to Germany in 2005 — a total of 504,000 tons of fish, crabs, molluscs and fish products — might well be contaminated despite inspections because only random samples are tested.

Now, another dye is causing a stir among the people of Hong Kong. Sudan Red — a synthetic *azo* dye that is soluble in oils, fats and waxes — was discovered in egg yolks. It is designed to color gasoline and shoe polish, for instance. Though the use of Sudan Red in food has been prohibited since 1995 in Europe because of its carcinogenic effects, the substance has been turning up in imported goods over and over again. It has been found, for example, in chili and paprika powders (in extreme cases up to as much as four grams per kilogram), as well as in tomatoes and products containing paprika.

The result is that Hong Kongers have lost faith in fish and eggs imported from mainland China, and such products have been boycotted. The public outrage is having an effect: Hong Kong is now helping China with its food quality control.

I try to get a feel for the situation by visiting the market in Hang Hau on Sunday. In one corner of the market hall, a grumpy lady is selling Chinese eggs at

Who Cloned My Cat? Fun Adventures in Biotechnology by R. Renneberg
Copyright © 2011 by Pan Stanford Publishing Pte Ltd
www.panstanford.com
978-981-4267-65-6

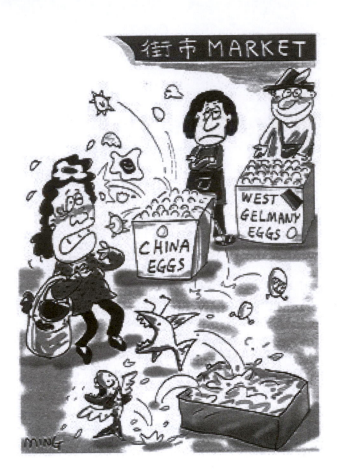

just 20 HK cents apiece; there's not a single customer around. (HK$0.20 is about 26 US-cents) A few meters away, a friendly egg-seller has got brown eggs at HK 60 cents each. His handwritten sign says in his best Chinglish: WEST GELMAN EGGS!

A Chinese friend informs me that after the war, there were two things synonymous with the highest quality products: *Made in Japan* and *Made in West Germany*. "And because we have trouble with the pronunciation of "R" and "L", the word becomes GELMAN!" she adds.

Now, my curiosity is getting the better of me! The grumpy woman's brown eggs don't seem to be that different from the top quality, expensive West Gelman ones. But wait a second! What was it again? Ah yes, since January 1st, 2004, German law requires that every egg be stamped with a special code — and this law applies throughout Europe. The code includes: cage specifications; country, state or province of origin; and the producer's code.

Now, let me check these eggs again... Aha! These West Gelman eggs don't have stamps! "I knew it!" says my Chinese friend with resignation, and lets out a sigh.

Chapter 67

DNA and My Ancestors

"Where do we come from?" The answer to this most ancient of humankind's questions was about to become my scientific New Year's present — to myself. Courtesy of biotech!

In the Genographic Project, an endeavor launched by the National Geographic Society in the US and supported by IBM, DNA samples from people around the world are being collected, analyzed and compared with historical DNA. For about 125 US dollars, *National Geographic* magazine is inviting the general public to take the DNA test. So, I filled out the Internet questionnaire and transferred the money.

A week later, the test kit arrived with a manual. First, I had to take a sample of my oral mucosa by scraping with two tiny brushes for five minutes. Then, I inserted the brushes containing my DNA sample into some small tubes and sent them by airmail to the US for analysis. The male Y-chromosome, passed from fathers to sons since time immemorial, would be scrutinized under a genetic microscope. An email arrived three days later with my personal code number, which would allow me to access my results. Another six weeks after that and my results were ready: the email subject said: *Ready! Check your results!*

I typed my code number excitedly into the Genographic Project website and a world map popped up on the screen. A red arrow started in Africa (Kenya and Ethiopia), then rushed north, passed over the Middle East, and stopped somewhere in the top-left of Greece. *Your Y-chromosome identifies you as member of Haplo group E3b (M35)*, said the computer. Aha!

Next, my precious male Y-chromosome was shown on the screen using STR (short tandem repeat) analysis. These are repeated DNA sequences that indicate mutation information. The 12 STRs showed my unique genetic profile.

Then, the analysis compared my DNA with that found in fossils. The starting point of my DNA (like all Eurasian males) was an "Adam" with the genetic marker M168 located in what is now Ethiopia around 31,000 to 79,000 years ago.

Who Cloned My Cat? Fun Adventures in Biotechnology by R. Renneberg
Copyright © 2011 by Pan Stanford Publishing Pte Ltd
www.panstanford.com
978-981-4267-65-6

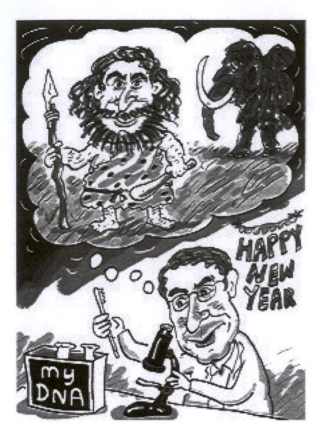

His nomadic descendants then moved north. This period is documented in my DNA as the so-called YAP mutation of the Y-chromosome, which was found in a prehistoric man who lived in northeast Africa about 50,000 years ago.

My next genetic marker was M35, typical for New Stone Age farmers from 20,000 years ago in the Middle East. According to the database, my particular E3b variation occurs mainly in southern and eastern parts of the Mediterranean Sea.

In fact, in my humble family tree, there is indeed a Greek church painter (regrettably, not very famous) — as well as a number of relatives in Transylvania and Hungary.

I suddenly hit upon a radical idea: we should be DNA-testing all of our xenophobic fellow citizens; they would be surprised to learn what they have in their German blood!

Any day now, we'll get the DNA results for a very charming Chinese lady whom I persuaded to take the same test. Women can even trace their DNA to the "mitochondrial Eve," who lived 150,000 to 170,000 years ago.

Where and when did her great great (etc.) grandmother and my great great (etc.) grandfather separate?

Find out what happens in the next chapter! In the meantime, I strongly recommend that you visit *www.nationalgeographic.com/genographic* and get your DNA tested! Maybe, without realizing it, we're related?

Chapter 68

The Chinese also Come from Africa

My 170 Chinese students looked at me in disbelief: I'd just told them where they come from — even the people of Beijing are descended from Africans. I had already told them about my own ancestors, and they were amused (see Chap. 67, *DNA and My Ancestors*, p. 147). But then the DNA result from my Chinese friend Claire arrived. Claire is Hong Kong's famous dolphin trainer (see Chap. 34, *Flipper Gets Artificially Fertilized*, p. 73).

Claire's DNA wasn't taken from the main chromosome of the cell nucleus (in my case, the male Y-chromosome) but from the genetic material of the cellular power plants, the mitochondria. She, like all females, can trace her DNA back to the "mitochondrial Eve" — the woman whose mitochondrial DNA (mtDNA) can be found in all living humans today. Only the female gamete, the ovum, contains mitochondria, not the sperm cells; mtDNA is handed down from mothers to daughters. However, the mitochondrial Eve was *not* the first woman and not the only one alive in her time; the mitochondrial hereditary lines from other women became extinct while those from "Eve" survived.

These are the principles behind the DNA migration map of the Genographic Project, initiated by the National Geographic Society. The analysis compared Claire's mtDNA with the Cambridge Reference Sequence (CRS), and she was included in the haplotype B group. Exactly 596 DNA letters of her mtDNA were analyzed for mutations. These DNA mutations were passed down from mothers to children, but only daughters handed them down to their daughters.

The first "trail" leads back 150,000 to 170,000 years to "Eve." The marker Eva-L1/L0 was found in East Africa before it spread north. Afterwards, L1 mutated into L2. L2 was found in West Africa, where it still dominates today, and most Afro-Americans belong to this group as well — a result of the slave trade. The next marker, L3, was found in a woman who was born in North Africa 80,000 years ago. Her group was the first to leave Africa.

But why did her group migrate? Well, blame the Ice Age! During the Ice Age in Africa, the drying climate was more of a problem than the cold, as huge masses

Who Cloned My Cat? Fun Adventures in Biotechnology **by R. Renneberg**
Copyright © 2011 by Pan Stanford Publishing Pte Ltd
www.panstanford.com
978-981-4267-65-6

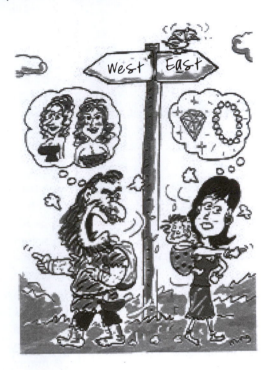

of water formed into ice. As the Ice Age receded, the climate then changed from dry to warm and humid.

At that time, *Homo sapiens* numbered around 10,000 and used stone tools and created Stone Age art. While the Sahara belt had become impassable during the Ice Age, it was transformed into a green savannah full of animals that could be hunted. This gateway to the north was open only for a short time, though; the Sahara would eventually become impenetrable once again.

Claire's (and my) nomadic ancestors followed the animal herds to the north. Intellectual abilities developed as well: language, planning and cooperation made the migration into new territories faster.

Next, they passed through Sinai in the eastern Mediterranean Sea region. They came into contact with Neanderthals during that time — but apparently not very close contact.

Some 10,000 years later, the great separation occurred of Claire's ancestors and mine. My haplo group N moved in the direction of Turkey and Greece while Claire's group with the marker B moved to the Central Asian steppe between the Caspian Sea and Lake Baikal — to Mongolia (and across the completely ice-covered Bering Strait to America) or India, then up to China or down to Polynesia.

It must have been in the Middle East where my male great great ancestors were abandoned by her female great great ancestors.

To make the parting easier, Claire's great great grandma probably said (in a mysterious language): "Don't worry! Our great great grandchildren will surely meet again in a few thousand years!" She was right — as women nearly always are!

Chapter 69

Tanking Up with Corn

PUT BIO IN YOUR TANK has become a popular slogan in China. The bio boom is a result of sharply rising oil and fuel prices. Suddenly, the oldest biotechnology in the world — the yeast fermentation of sugars into alcohol — is being heralded as the savior of the future.

China has been subsidizing biofuels since 2002, which has meant producing ethanol mainly from corn, sweet potato and beet. According to the official *Xinhua* news agency, one fifth of all cars in China use bioethanol. And not too long ago, it was announced that biodiesel produced from animal and vegetable fats would be available at Chinese gas stations. All these measures could help reduce the increasingly intolerable air pollution in China and reduce the country's dependence on oil.

But not everyone is so optimistic. "Put *hunger* in your tank," some critics have said, arguing that limited arable land and the world's poor grain harvest over the past years are exacerbating the problem.

Grain prices have risen steeply over the past few months, and continuing to produce alcohol from food could set prices spiraling out of control, leading to social instability and unrest. The Chinese government has now applied the emergency brakes: bioethanol producers now require a license — and acquiring one can be a complicated process.

China is setting trends that many other countries could follow. By 2020, the EU plans for 20 percent of all its energy needs to come from agricultural production. In 2004, 34 million tons of grain were turned into ethanol in the US alone — all of which was, of course, heavily subsidized by the government. Corn-importing countries such as Japan, Mexico and Egypt are even worried about a possible decrease in US exports, which make up 70 percent of world trade.

Another point critics often make is the lack of efficiency of biofuel programs. Brazil seems to be the only country that gets more energy out of sugarcane than it puts in because it also ferments byproducts like crushed pulp. India and China, by contrast, cannot produce sufficient amounts of corn or sugarcane for ethanol

Who Cloned My Cat? Fun Adventures in Biotechnology **by R. Renneberg**
Copyright © 2011 by Pan Stanford Publishing Pte Ltd
www.panstanford.com
978-981-4267-65-6

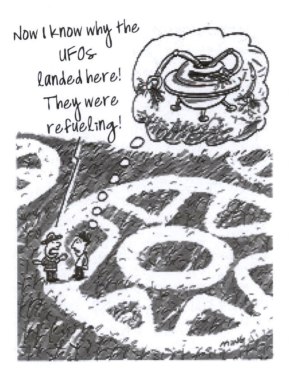

Now I know why the UFOs landed here! They were refueling!

production due to their small-scale farming practices as well as shortages of fertilizer. Another problem, which no one has yet talked about, is the precious water that will be needed to irrigate the fields.

Help could come through the use of a broader range of resources: straw, wood, liquid manure, waste, and also special "energy plants." Biotechnologists are busy developing energy-rich crops such as corn with higher starch content and with optimized enzymes and microorganisms that accelerate ethanol production. Methods that allow the use of plant substrates or agricultural waste, including the use of cellulose, are also being developed.

One area of consideration is that of genetically modified energy plants that can grow in deserts.

Professor Alan MacDiarmid (University of Texas at Dallas and University of Pennsylvania), winner of the Nobel Prize for Chemistry in 2000, recently gave a lecture about agri-energy at my university in Hong Kong. Showing a picture of an angry-looking US President Bush, he declared, "Oil cravings make you aggressive!" — to the amusement of the attending Chinese students.

MacDiarmid had just set up a research center in China that looks into the country's supply of bioenergy. In the vast desert areas of the west of the country, hardy, energy-supplying plants — which do not compete with food crops — could be grown and at the same time provide poor farmers with much-needed income. Indeed, contented Chinese farmers are important for peace and stability both within the country and outside. Will MacDiarmid's ideas work?*

Read more on this subject in Chap. 79, *Biofuel from Wood?* p. 175.

---

* Sadly, Alan MacDiarmid passed away in 2007.

Chapter 70

Competition Is Good for Business

"We women have to believe in ourselves, or no one else will."

Rosalyn Sussman Yalow lived by this motto her whole life. She believed that the world could not afford to waste half of its talent. But achieving success in science was a tall order for a Jewish woman in 1930s' America. Discrimination was routine in every sector — and academia was no exception.

By the late 1930s' when Rosalyn Sussman attended college, nuclear physics was one of science's most exciting fields. Rosalyn had already begun planning her career as a physicist. In January 1941, New York's Hunter College would make her their first woman to receive a Bachelor's degree. Yet a career at a university was still unthinkable, and as a compromise one of her physics professors offered her a job as a part-time secretary.

The turning point came as the US entered World War II, and the paucity of male students at universities gave her the opportunity to work as an assistant at the University of Illinois at Urbana. When she transferred there in September 1941, she was the only woman among 400 participants at the first meeting. One of her colleagues once commented sarcastically, "Well, competition is good for business."

In Urbana, Rosalyn met the physics student Aaron Yalow, whom she married in 1943, two years before obtaining her doctoral degree. From 1950, she worked for the Veterans Administration Hospital in New York. Alongside her obligations as a mother of two, she took an active role in a research team under one Dr. Solomon A. Berson.

As so often in science, her great discovery was something of a byproduct of her work. A certain Dr. Mirsky believed that diabetes arose through the enzymatic degradation of insulin. This is what Rosalyn Yalow wanted to test. Diabetic and non-diabetic subjects were first given pig insulin and then intravenously injected with radioactively marked insulin. As the radioactive insulin had a much slower rate of disappearance from the plasma of the diabetics than that of the non-diabetics, Yalow and Berson postulated that antibodies formed in the diabetics' blood against the animal insulin and therefore bound to the radioactive insulin. The

Who Cloned My Cat? Fun Adventures in Biotechnology by R. Renneberg
Copyright © 2011 by Pan Stanford Publishing Pte Ltd
www.panstanford.com
978-981-4267-65-6

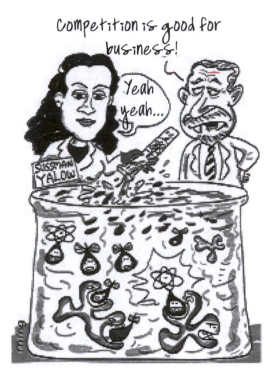

work went so much against the widely held beliefs of the mid-1950s that the *Journal of Clinical Investigation* only accepted it for publication after a long, drawn-out struggle.

Next came the brilliant idea. A defined number of antibodies against insulin and later a known amount of radioactive insulin were added to a test tube containing an unknown concentration of insulin. The natural insulin and the radioactive insulin "competed" to bind to the antibodies. As a result, the amount of bound radioactive insulin could be used to measure the amount of existing natural insulin: the more radioactive insulin that was measured, the less natural insulin there was in the solution. "Competition is good for business," indeed!

The radioimmunoassay (RIA) had been born! The procedure allowed the measurement of substances in extremely low concentrations.

In 1977, Rosalyn Yalow became only the second woman in history to be awarded the Nobel Prize in Medicine, for her work in using RIA to classify peptide hormones. Before her, Gerty Theresa Cori (1896–1957) with her husband Carl F. Cori (1896–1984) received the Prize for their work on enzymes from animal tissues. And since the Nobel Prize cannot be awarded posthumously, the contribution of Solomon Berson, who had passed away by that time, went unrecognized.

The irony of this story is that Yalow and Berson's paper mentioned above has become one of the journal's most frequently cited. To laughter from the audience attending her Nobel presentation, Rosalyn Yalow showed off the first rejection letter from the journal.

In fact, I just received one of those rejection letters from London's *Nature Methods*. How annoying! Unfortunately, getting a rejection letter from *Nature* is no guarantee that you'll end up with a Nobel Prize.

Chapter 71

Amino Acids, not Made in Japan!

In the summer of 1973 in Hannover, Prof. Karl Schügerl gave Christian Wandrey the best advice he had ever been given: "As a chemist, why don't you do something totally different and study biotechnology under Prof. Kula?"

Maria-Regina Kula was already an authority on biotechnology at that time. My friend Christian Wandrey told me his story when we met in Hong Kong: "I met her in a motorway restaurant somewhere between Hannover and Braunschweig — to make things as convenient and efficient as possible. I went because I had been urged to do so, but I didn't expect much to come out of it." However, the meeting would have far-reaching consequences.

Wandrey eventually visited Prof. Kula's lab, where a membrane was being used as a molecular filter to separate out enzymes so they could be reused in a "reactor." Wandrey thought to himself: If a membrane can be use to filter thick enzymes and fine dirt can be flushed away through the pores, then raw material can also be processed using enzymes. Its products can be filtered by the membrane and the enzyme can be reused again *in situ*! The enzyme membrane reactor (EMR) was born. The prototype is located in the Deutsches Museum among the "100 most important technological inventions."

In 1979, Wandrey, who had just received his PhD, was sitting on the train with Prof. Kula, sipping coffee on the way back from a conference on biotechnology. They were discussing how, in order to produce amino acids, some enzymes require additional compounds, such as the cofactor $NADH_2$ — which cost a fortune at that time. Wandrey stirred his coffee, deep in thought. Finally, he said, "What about regenerating the cofactor?"

Professor Kula told Wandrey that this could The radioimmunoassay (RIA) had been born! be achieved very easily. In fact, she told him, his colleague Herman Sahm at Jülich Research Center had just discovered formate dehydrogenase (FDH) in yeast. FDH produces active hydrogen in the form of NADH and CO_2, and the gaseous CO_2 is released from the reaction. And the substrate of FDH, formic acid, was dirt cheap to produce. The reaction was quickly scribbled on a napkin.

Who Cloned My Cat? Fun Adventures in Biotechnology by R. Renneberg
Copyright © 2011 by Pan Stanford Publishing Pte Ltd
www.panstanford.com
978-981-4267-65-6

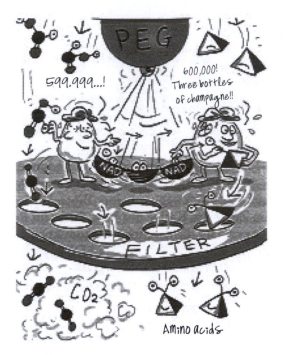

In the laboratory, the active enzymes were isolated together with FDH in an EMR to produce amino acids. Formic acid and other inexpensive materials were used. Everything was going well — except for the tiny NAD molecules. They kept passing through the membrane along with the product and needed to be replaced rather than regenerated. It was necessary to increase their molecular weight considerably without affecting their solubility in water. The solution to the problem came from the late Braunschweig biochemist Frits Bückmann. He successfully bound NAD^+ to polyethylene glycol (PEG) molecules, which are 100 times bigger in size and completely soluble in water. Picture NAD like a pendulum, tied by a rope to a giant rock (PEG).

The following is what happens in an EMR. The NAD-pendulum is loaded with two hydrogen atoms by the FDH. It swings to the amino acid dehydrogenase, which picks up the two hydrogens and uses them for synthesis. The "empty" pendulum swings back to the FDH, and the process repeats.

Wandrey's students in Jülich reported that they were able to use the coenzyme pendulum 10,000 times. Wandrey promised a bottle of (German) sparkling wine to the student who managed 100,000 cycles. "How about a bottle of *real* champagne for 200,000 cycles?" asked one smart female doctoral student. After 600,000 cycles, Wandrey ended up having to pay for three French bottles.

In 1981, the first EMR was launched by the Degussa company in Konstanz, Germany. In 2005, a Degussa EMR plant was opened in Nanning, China with an annual production capacity of 500 tons of L-methionine. A sign outside reads: EMR FROM JÜRICH (GERMANY). "Jürich" is the Chinese version of the German "Jülich".

Even the Japanese, the kings of amino acid production from glutamate to lysine (see Chap. 9, *007 and the Soup Stock*, p. 17), are importing special amino acids from Germany. In Japan and China, at any rate, Christian Wandrey is a big hero.

Chapter 72

Busy Bees: It's All in Their Genes!

Honeybees (*Apis mellifera*) are amazing insects. They communicate direction and distance to their food source through a waggle dance, a discovery that earned Karl von Frisch (1886–1982) from Austria a Nobel Prize in 1971.

But what mechanisms govern reproduction, division of labor and social has coexistence among bees? Fifty years after he decoded DNA structures, the great James Watson was asked: "If you could start a new career as a scientist…?" He answered: "…then I would work on the connection between genes and behavior."

The genetic code of the honeybee was completely sequenced in October 2006. Now, scientists are looking for the genetic "program" for their social life — if such a thing exists.

Norwegian Gro V. Amdam has been fascinated by bees and ants since her childhood. She now works in the US and presented the first comprehensive study looking at the genetic and hormonal regulation of complex social behavior by a single gene using honeybees as a model organism. Naturally, the media were all over this stylish scientist with blue eyes and blond locks.

Everything is arranged and regulated in the bees' universe: the role a given bee plays depends on its gender, age and "caste." The queen and the (male) drone bees concern themselves only with reproduction while all the other bees have to carry out various work-related tasks. Workers start out as nurse bees that care for larvae in the nest. Later, at the age of three weeks, they embark on foraging trips, specializing in either pollen or nectar collection.

Such activities seem to be determined by the protein vitellogenin. Vitellogenin is involved in egg production in all egg-laying animals and is an essential factor in good egg development. It is peculiar that this protein can be found in worker bees, which are essentially sterile. It is also known that nectar collectors have less vitellogenin than pollen collectors have.

Scientists can now use RNA interference (as already discussed; see Chap. 32, *The Gene Off Switch*, p. 69) to "knock down" the vitellogenin gene, thereby affecting normal protein production.

Who Cloned My Cat? Fun Adventures in Biotechnology by R. Renneberg
Copyright © 2011 by Pan Stanford Publishing Pte Ltd
www.panstanford.com
978-981-4267-65-6

When the expression of vitellogenin is suppressed via RNAi, the affected bees show reduced levels of vitellogenin in their hemolymph — the bee's equivalent of blood. At the same time, they also have high levels of juvenile hormones, which is typical for foragers. Tests have shown clearly that "knocked-down" bees become foragers earlier and prefer collecting nectar, but they also live shorter lives than normal bees do. It is believed that honeybee vitellogenin scavenges free radicals, acting as an antioxidant shield and thereby increasing longevity. According to Gro Amdam, vitellogenin coordinates three core aspects of the social life of bees: it paces the onset of foraging behavior, primes bees for specialized foraging tasks, and enhances longevity.

Lowering vitellogenin levels makes bees leave the nest earlier to look for food and return with nectar instead of pollen — both to the beekeeper's delight.

Efforts are now geared towards studying vitellogenin in other insects. The fruit fly *Drosophila* (see Chap. 13, *Vitamin C and the Fly*, p. 27) also has vitellogenin

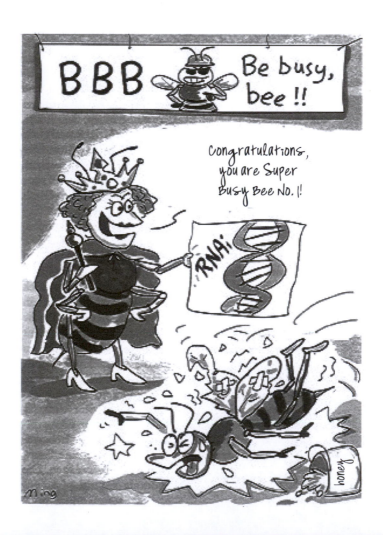

in its hemolymph. However, a fruit fly is a non-social insect that lives a solitary life and collects food only for itself.

It seems that, in the bee's case, evolution — ingeniously lazy as it is — has employed a preexisting mechanism from other insects for a new function. Very economical!

And what can we conclude from all this? Mother Nature rewards "smart laziness"!

Chapter 73

Leeuwenhoek's Wee Beasties

Antonie van Leeuwenhoek (1632–1723) opened up a whole new world on September 17, 1683 in Delft, the Netherlands, when he described the deposits on his teeth under a microscope. A merchant and self-taught scientist, Leeuwenhoek (1632–1723) became the first person to see bacteria and sketch them.

It all began when Leeuwenhoek observed a spectacle maker grind lenses at a fair. He soon learned how to do it himself and his quest to make ever-stronger lenses would become an obsession. One day, Leeuwenhoek hit upon the idea of studying a drop of water from his rain barrel. He got the most terrible shock when he looked at it under his microscope: it was teeming with tiny creatures, swimming about as if they were playing with one another! Leeuwenhoek estimated them to be a thousand times smaller than the size of the eye of a louse.

Encouraged by a friend, in 1673, Leeuwenhoek wrote an enthusiastic letter in Dutch to what was then the most prestigious scientific organization, the Royal Society of London. The learned gentlemen were most surprised to read a description of "cavorting wee beasties," as Leeuwenhoek chose to call them in his letter. The scientists of the Royal Society were skeptical — microscopically small creatures? Having never attended a university, Leeuwenhoek didn't have the credentials to sway the Englishmen. Unconvinced that these were really living creatures, the British sent a commission to Delft to see the "beasties" with their own eyes. And they were soon very excited about the findings.

After being unanimously voted in as a member, Leeuwenhoek sent some 560 letters to the Royal Society in 1680. The Queen of England, King Frederick I of Prussia as well as the Russian Tsar Peter the Great (who had come to the Netherlands under a false name to study the art of shipbuilding) all paid him a visit.

Until recently, modern scientists had also been puzzled by Leeuwenhoek's discovery: could he really have seen bacteria by using only a single lens? British scientific publisher Brian Ford wanted to know for sure and dug into the Royal

Who Cloned My Cat? Fun Adventures in Biotechnology by R. Renneberg
Copyright © 2011 by Pan Stanford Publishing Pte Ltd
www.panstanford.com
978-981-4267-65-6

Society's archives. To his delight, he found Leeuwenhoek's letters carefully archived. Both of his microscopes and hundreds of his preparations were found in nine packages, wrapped four times in stiff paper and well preserved for over three centuries!

It was a scientific gold mine. Ford began some experiments. He studied the samples using a modern electron microscope and what he saw were perfectly prepared specimens! The authenticity of Leeuwenhoek's various scientific discoveries was completely verifiable: infusoria in 1674, bacteria in 1676, spermatozoa in 1677, and the banded pattern of muscle fibers in 1682. Detailed pictures of spirally twisted bacteria (*spirilla*) and blood corpuscles can be seen on Ford's website (*www.brianjford.com/wav-spd.htm*) — just as the master saw them.

The curious Leeuwenhoek had achieved, through his skill, inquisitiveness and persistence, far more than many of his academic contemporaries — who, if asked how many teeth a donkey had, would have preferred to look for the answer in Aristotle's writings rather than actually look into a donkey's mouth!

Leeuwenhoek's tiny bugs were a fascinating novelty for quite some time but were eventually forgotten. Nobody imagined that the "cavorting wee beasties" would be responsible for horrific and disastrous plagues — not to mention crispy bread, finely brewed beers, premium wines, and delicious cheeses!

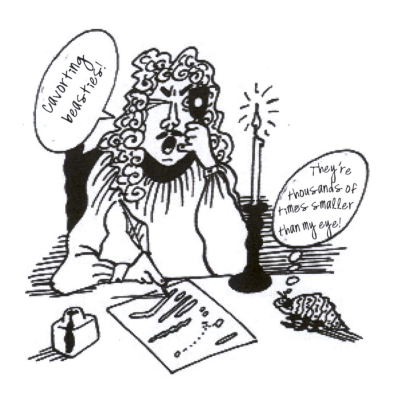

Chapter 74

Genetic Engineering in Your Washer

"Lennebelg-san, gomen nasai… Boil wash programs? We never boil our laundry… We use *baioteku*: good old *koso pauwa*!" This is what Michiro, wife of the famous Prof. Saburo Fukui, told me when I was invited to Kyoto in the 1980s. No wonder I couldn't find the boil wash program on the washing machine — even with the help of my dictionary. Here, *koso pauwa* (enzyme power) is the magic word for laundry care. In Japan, people only ever wash their laundry using lukewarm water.

Today, "koso pauwa" can be found in many detergents all over the world as well (see Chap. 12, *"Irashaimase, Baioteku"*, p. 25; Chap. 24, *A Tale About a Cold*, p. 51 and Chap. 45, *Molecular Laundresses*, p. 95). These enzymes are mostly genetically manipulated, and, in every sense of the word, they "cauterize" — detergents, softeners and bleaches are not unaggressive substances.

One single enzyme started it all: subtilisin. It was discovered in Copenhagen by Kaj Ulrik Linderstrøem-Lang (1896–1959) in 1947 in a bacterium called *Bacillus subtilis*. This longtime director of the Carlsberg brewery's research laboratory was not only a fantastic scientist but also a courageous activist in the resistance movement against the Nazis. Denmark was occupied from 1940 to 1943.

Subtilisin is produced by the bacteria in order to cut down big foreign food proteins. Bacteria have no "mouths" and can only take up food proteins if they are first split into single building blocks (amino acids). The bacteria are cultivated in giant bioreactors, yielding the enzyme by the ton. Subtilisin contains 275 amino acids. With the help of water molecules, it breaks down other proteins into amino acids. Amazingly, the protease remains undamaged in the process.

Stains that contain proteins like egg yolk, blood, milk or sweat act like glue in fabrics. At high temperatures, the protein curdles on the textile fibers and is even harder to remove. Subtilisin breaks down this "glue" into small particles and allows dirt to be flushed out. This energy-saving process takes place in lukewarm water; boiling water destroys the enzymes instead.

Unfortunately, in the presence of bleaching agents, subtilisin loses about 80 percent of its activity. To counter this, in the early 1990s, the enzyme was

Who Cloned My Cat? Fun Adventures in Biotechnology **by R. Renneberg**
Copyright © 2011 by Pan Stanford Publishing Pte Ltd
www.panstanford.com
978-981-4267-65-6

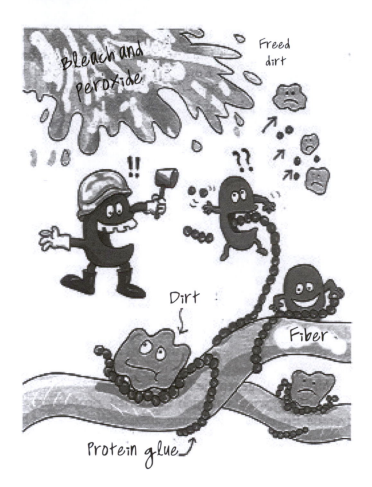

genetically modified by the US company Genentech (today, Genencor) in San Francisco, California. Protein engineers compared the 3D structure of native (non-oxidized) subtilisin with that incubated with hydrogen peroxide. One extra oxygen was visible on the sulfur atom of methionine at position 222. The oxygen seems to be the reason for the loss of catalytic efficiency of the amino acid. When methionine was replaced by one of the other 19 amino acids, the success was overwhelming: all the new mutant enzymes were more stable than the wild-type enzyme.

It is estimated that nowadays hundreds of tons of genetically modified enzymes are produced every year. Not only proteases but also starch-dissolving amylases are genetically stabilized. Consumers aren't complaining. I'm quite sure that all those opponents of gene technology have already found their "bitter enemies" in their washing machines.

But the small quantities of enzymes found in bio-detergents are without doubt harmless to humans and the environment. On the contrary, they have reduced energy requirements and the raw materials needed more than tenfold. That's reason enough to give a respectful, Japanese-style bow to the genetic engineers!

Chapter 75

Yams and Cortisone

On June 8, 1951, a telegram was sent to Dr. Carl Djerassi and his tiny company Syntex. Tadeusz Reichstein (the discoverer of vitamin C synthesis; see Chap. 13, *Vitamin C and the Fly*, p. 27), who had just won the Nobel Prize a year earlier, had compared Djerassi's synthesized cortisone with that isolated from adrenal glands and confirmed its authenticity. Djerassi jumped for joy. The Mexican company belonging to the 34-year-old Djerassi had won the worldwide race to synthesize cortisone.

In the early 1930s, Reichstein and Edward C. Kendall (1886–1972) isolated cortisone (a steroid hormone) from adrenal glands of animals and for their work received the 1950 Nobel Prize for Physiology or Medicine along with Philip S. Hench. About a year later, it was discovered that cortisone could relieve pain in arthritis sufferers. Given the high demand, it was clear that a chemical synthesis needed to be found. But the complicated production process involving some 36 steps drove the price to nearly 200 US dollars per gram.

Carl Djerassi grew up in pre-war Vienna and fled the Nazis in 1938. Despite arriving penniless in New York at the age of 16, he managed to graduate as a chemist. His small Mexican company Syntex succeeded in extracting the steroid diosgenin from wild inedible yams. The natives of Mexico and Central America had long used roots of yams both for washing laundry and for killing fish. Djerassi transformed diosgenin chemically into the female sex hormone progesterone and later into the male sex hormone testosterone. He was in competition with the world's greatest chemists in the race to chemically produce cortisone.

Djerassi couldn't enjoy his success for long. Soon after, he received an inquiry from the Upjohn Company of Kalamazoo in Michigan to supply 10 tons of progesterone. Since the world's entire annual production at that time was probably less than one-hundredth that amount, such a request seemed outlandish. He concluded that Upjohn had found a way to synthesize cortisone using progesterone as a chemical intermediary — rather than using it as a therapeutic hormone.

The conclusion proved correct when, a few weeks later, a patent was issued to Upjohn. Two of its scientists, Durey H. Peterson and Herbert C. Murray, had made

Who Cloned My Cat? Fun Adventures in Biotechnology by R. Renneberg
Copyright © 2011 by Pan Stanford Publishing Pte Ltd
www.panstanford.com
978-981-4267-65-6

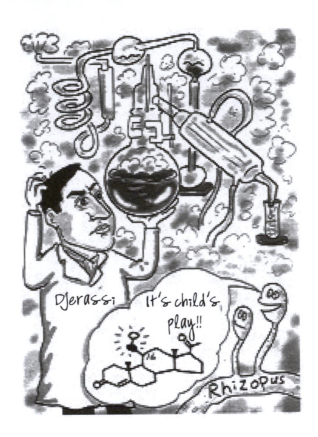

a sensational discovery: the fermentation of progesterone with the fungus *Rhizopus arrhizus* resulting in a key, one-step transformation on the way to cortisone. With the help of the fungus, the 36 synthesis steps could be reduced to just 11. The price of cortisone dropped to 7 US dollars per gram, and by 1980, after further advances, to below 1 US dollar.

The cortisone example (and before that, vitamin C) has proved that biotechnology and chemistry cannot be separated from each other. The combination of both biological and chemical processes will grow hugely over the next decade. Microbes or their enzymes can accomplish these targeted syntheses, which with pure chemical synthesis would be too expensive and complicated.

A few months later, Djerassi found solace by synthesizing, with Georg Rosenkranz and Luis E. Miramontes, the progestin norethindrone, the first oral contraceptive for women. Djerassi became the "Father of the Pill" in 1957 and thus a millionaire, art collector (with a great Paul Klee collection) and patron of the arts. Now 86, he is hard at work on his second career: writing thrilling novels about scientists — which he calls "science-in-fiction." I have devoured all of them. Carl visited me in Hong Kong recently. He is full of energy and very charismatic. One of my idols!

After the English language edition of my recent book came out (*Biotechnology for Beginners*, Academic Press, 2008), Djerassi sent me an Austrian postage stamp bearing his portrait with Vienna in the background and the words: *Carl Djerassi, chemist/novelist: born 1923, expelled 1938, reconciled 2003.*

Chapter 76

Xylophagy in My Bookcase

Never heard of xylophagy before? Me neither, until one day I opened the drawer of my bookcase and, instead of my old manuscripts, it was filled with brown pulp. The university accommodations office flew into a panic and on the very same day had the bookcase removed from the wall and sprayed with a strong pesticide.

I had nothing against them doing it; during a half-year absence, one of my Chinese colleagues had his entire apartment affected by xylophagy. *Xylon* is the Greek for wood; xylophagy refers to the consumption of wood.

Termites belong to such wood consumers. They themselves are unable to break down wood and digest it, but their guts contain flagellates and bacteria that are their symbiotic wood-degraders. This highly effective miniature bio-factory produces enough energy for survival. Cellulase is the special enzyme that can break down cellulose, one major component of wood. The waste product of this process is (relatively) large amounts of carbon dioxide, carbon monoxide, hydrogen and methane.

Termites, incidentally, are the biggest biological producers of methane gas. Methane is a highly active greenhouse gas. Other methane-producing culprits are ruminants, especially domestic cattle. They also carry cellulase microbes in their intestines. Without them, neither termites nor cattle could digest cellulose. Interestingly, the mammoth also produced methane. After hunting drove it to extinction, the temperature of the Earth dropped, and the Ice Age intensified!

Meanwhile, the US Department of Energy is showing an interest in cellulase. Some 385 million US dollars have been invested in a project to transform cellulose into ethanol — one way of producing biofuel (see Chap. 69, *Tanking Up with Corn*, p. 151) without using food products and thus competing with the production of food for consumption, such as corn.

The sought-after enzyme is an old acquaintance of the Americans. After the Japanese attacked Pearl Harbor, America joined WWII, and from the very beginning of the war in the Pacific, the US had to fight microbial enemies as well. In the tropical battlefield, the US Army's cellulose-containing equipment disintegrated

Who Cloned My Cat? Fun Adventures in Biotechnology by R. Renneberg
Copyright © 2011 by Pan Stanford Publishing Pte Ltd
www.panstanford.com
978-981-4267-65-6

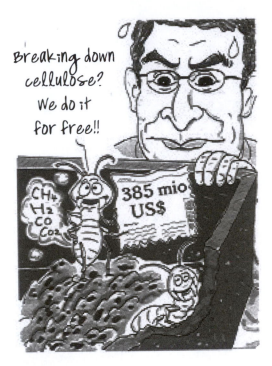

Breaking down cellulose? We do it for free!!

CH₄ H₂ CO CO₂

385 mio. US$

with frightening speed. The culprit was the cellulase-producing fungus *Trichoderma viride*, found in New Guinea on a rotten cartridge belt made from cotton. The fungus, which is now named *Trichoderma reesei* after the eminent American cellulose researcher Elwyn T. Reese, secretes cellulases extracellularly. Cellulose is thus broken down into sugar, which is a food source for the fungus.

Although the price per ton of dry lignocellulosic biomass is considerably lower than that of grain starch, when it comes to conversion into sugar, it simply cannot compete. The firm structure of cellulose, vital for plants, is a major obstacle. The crystalline cellulose is bound to hemicellulose and lignin, and isn't water-soluble. Most microbes, therefore, are unable to break down wood without enzymatic pre-treatment.

The biotech process has remained uneconomical: after 30 days in a bioreactor, even the most efficient lignin-degrading fungus leaves 40 percent of the lignin intact. Pre-treating lignocellulose with acid is necessary to ensure efficient enzymatic breakdown — and the removal of the acid is an expensive business. The cost could be reduced by using steam or freeze explosion technologies with liquid ammonia to remove the acid. Another problem concerns the comparatively low activity of cellulases. Protein engineering might be a way of solving this — just as has been done with detergent enzymes (see Chap. 45, *Molecular Laundresses*, p. 95 and Chap. 74, *Genetic Engineering in Your Washer*, p. 163).

When I wrote to one of my German colleagues about my termite problem, he replied, "For goodness' sake, don't kill them! Send me a box of termites for my next visit to the German Tax Office!"

Chapter 77

DNA Gunshots into the Sea

"Kleg Wentel 4pm in HKU!" said the cryptic e-mail sent by my Chinese students on December 16, 2004.

"What is this!?" I wondered. Later, after asking around, I found out that everyone was going on a pilgrimage to the neighboring university to catch a glimpse of the golden boy of DNA research, J. Craig Venter — pioneer of genetic engineering, multimillionaire and world sailor. The American was responsible for dramatically accelerating the race to unlock the mysteries of the human genome with his privately funded for-profit project facing off against the government-funded Human Genome Project conducted by Francis Collins. The objective of his company Celera was simple: to patent the human genome.

His plans were shelved at the eleventh hour. On July 26, 2000 then-President Bill Clinton made an emphatic joint announcement arm in arm with Collins and Venter in seeming harmony: "Today, we are learning the language in which God created life."

At the time, Venter must surely have been both the most loathed and admired DNA researcher in the US. Still, there's no doubt that it was his involvement that sped up the sequencing of the human genome by years. For a while after, little was heard from him, but Venter is now once again back in the spotlight — which he loves so much.

The passionate sailor reported his latest coup from the Sargasso Sea in the Public Library of Science magazine *PLoS Biology* (*http://collections.plos.org/plosbiology/gos-2007.php*).

After his financial success with the DNA project, the millionaire bought himself a 90-foot yacht called *Sorcerer II* and, in the summer of 2002, went on a test voyage with his crew to the Sargasso Sea near the Bermuda Islands. The Sargasso Sea is where European eel spawn and is known as the biological "desert" of the ocean.

His expedition yielded astonishing results. The first six samples alone revealed more than 1.2 million new genes — almost 10 times as many as were known worldwide at that time. The "catch" included 782 photoreceptor genes,

Who Cloned My Cat? Fun Adventures in Biotechnology by R. Renneberg
Copyright © 2011 by Pan Stanford Publishing Pte Ltd
www.panstanford.com
978-981-4267-65-6

which code for enzymes that enable microscopic organisms to turn sunlight into energy. In addition, 50,000 genes capable of processing hydrogen were found. "Energy from sunlight and water hasn't been a very successful endeavor until now — this could change soon!" said Venter.

Instead of following the usual procedure of growing individual microbial cultures, the researchers fed the gene mix into their DNA sequencing machines back home — the entire genetic material, filtered out of 1500 liters of water. The result was 70,000 genes that were completely unknown.

It was possible to piece together complete gene sequences (genomes) of entire organisms; the samples contained at least 1800 species. Although the Sargasso Sea is considered one of the most extensively analyzed regions in the ocean, Venter discovered 148 totally unknown kinds of bacteria. Specialized computer software could then compare the new sequences against databases of information on genes with known functions. Chance favors the prepared mind!

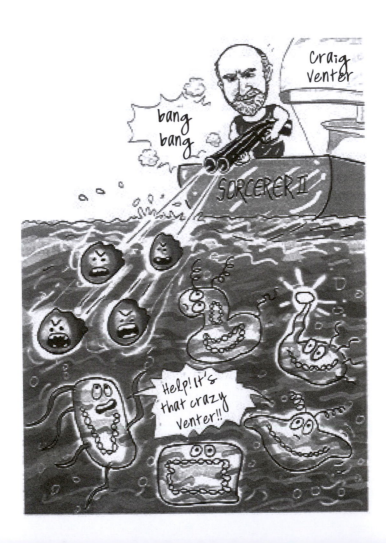

By using the highly automated gene technology to answer ecological questions, Venter has initiated a completely new research discipline: ecological metagenomics. Increasingly, biologists and geneticists, in particular, are homing in on the gene pool of entire ecosystems.

Sorcerer II sailed from the North Atlantic through the Panama Canal and ended its journey in the South Pacific. No less than the great Charles Darwin once traveled part of this route with H.M.S. *Beagle* and H.M.S. *Challenger*. Venter's journey, with commentary by the master himself, can be found at *www.sorcerer2expedition.org*.

For this latest venture, Venter once again used his "shotgun sequencing" approach that competed so impressively against the methods of the Human Genome Project. In this approach, DNA is broken up randomly into numerous small segments and sequenced. Several rounds of fragmentation and sequencing result in multiple overlapping segments, and software programs can then use the overlapping ends of different segments to assemble continuous sequences.

The ocean is a veritable goldmine for discoverers and scientists. Venter is already planning his next metagenome project: the air over New York. What could be floating or swarming there? Just imagine a metagenome comparison (sponsored by the EU!) of Venter's New York air with the world-renowned air over Berlin. Paul Linckes' brass band can accompany the project with their famous hit:

"Das ist die Berliner Luft Luft Luft,
so mit ihrem holden Duft Duft Duft,
wo nur selten was verpufft pufft pufft,
in dem Duft Duft Duft
dieser Luft Luft Luft.

Ja ja ja: Das ist…"

(Translation: *"That is the Berlin air air air,*
with its lovely scent scent scent,
it is where things seldom wither wither wither,
in the scent
of this air.

Yes yes yes: That is…")

Well, this could go on endlessly. Please continue reading instead!

Chapter 78

Genetic Fingerprints

In 1983, 15-year-old Lynda Mann was found raped and strangled in the village of Narborough, England. Three years later, Dawn Ashworth, also 15, was found in nearby Enderby. Police found no evidence. It was around this time that Alec Jeffreys, genetic scientist at the University of Leicester, England, published his restriction fragment length polymorphisms (RFLP) method — commonly pronounced "rif lip."

Doctor Jeffreys was investigating the evolution of a gene for myoglobin, the protein responsible for oxygen transport in muscles. After gel electrophoresis, he photographed the relevant DNA fragments. At 9am on September 15, 1984 he looked at the freshly developed images in the university darkroom. It showed DNA in various bands, resembling a product bar code. "Gosh," he thought, "what have we got here? Such varied patterns — each one very unique. It should be possible to distinguish different individuals with these!" Just a few hours later, Jeffreys and his team would coin the term "genetic fingerprinting" for their fortuitous discovery.

With Jeffreys' help, DNA from sperm traces at the crime scene was isolated and the DNA profile of the murderer was established. Then 5000 men between 16 and 34, who did not have alibis, were asked to give blood samples. Of course, the police did not expect the killer to come forward of his own accord. But they got a lead when, in August 1987, a woman told police that in the pub one day one of her colleagues had said that he'd helped a friend by providing a blood sample on his behalf. When police questioned the man, he told them that his friend, 27-year-old Colin Pitchfork, had convinced him he couldn't take the test because he'd already helped out someone else who was in trouble. But the truth was that Pitchfork was the killer. In January 1988, he pleaded guilty and received a life sentence.

Earlier, a mentally ill man had been released because his DNA did not match that of the sperm found at the crime scene. It was the first time in history that suspects had been convicted — and freed — on the basis of DNA analysis. Thanks DNA!

Who Cloned My Cat? Fun Adventures in Biotechnology **by R. Renneberg**
Copyright © 2011 by Pan Stanford Publishing Pte Ltd
www.panstanford.com
978-981-4267-65-6

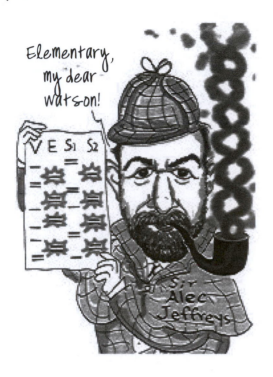

By 1987, DNA test results had become officially admissible as evidence in the US and the UK. Testing showed that neither eyewitnesses nor even the US Court of Justice are always reliable.

In *The Innocence Project*, New York defense lawyer Barry Scheck calls DNA "the gold standard of innocence." Since 1992, he has managed to release 201 innocent prisoners. Scheck has suggested that at least one in seven people sentenced to death is innocent!

More spectacular cases followed. Bones of the last Russian Tsar and his family were found and identified. DNA testing confirmed the identity of Josef Mengele, the notorious Auschwitz doctor — though, unfortunately, only after his fatal accident. The murderer of the German fashion icon Rudolph Moshammer was apprehended using DNA evidence.

After DNA matches put the suspect at the scene, the assassin of the Swedish foreign secretary Anna Lindh was convicted. DNA paternity tests have also increasingly become the norm.

Alec J. Jeffreys was knighted in 1994, and he is repeatedly nominated for the Nobel Prize. Great Britain, for one, is proud of its four million DNA fingerprints in the police database. Sir Alec has opposed the use of DNA profiling, however: "No criminalization! We should gather the genetic fingerprints of all British people in a database, which should not be controlled by government. Then, without exception, everybody is treated equally." But who really believes that's true?

Sir Alec has been called the "DNA Sherlock Holmes." Holmes, of course, always has his loyal Dr. Watson by his side, and strangely enough, one of the co-discoverers of DNA structure has the same name: Dr. James Watson!

Chapter 79

Biofuel from Wood?

My friend and colleague Prof. Oreste Ghisalba from Basel dampened my optimism some years ago: bio is not always good! His argument was based on a study supported by the Swiss Federal Agencies of Energy, Environment and Agriculture on the ecological record of various biofuels. It showed that biofuels from rapeseed, rye, corn and soy are more harmful than they are useful.

The Swiss Federal Laboratories for Materials Testing and Research (Empa) in St. Gallen analyzed the whole biofuel cycle — from production through distribution to consumption. The tests scrutinized bioethanol and biomethanol as alternatives for gasoline, biomethane for natural gas, and of course biodiesel. Though they did indeed produce a lot less CO_2 during consumption, soil contamination due to intensive fertilization was a serious problem. In addition, nitrogen fertilizer produces the greenhouse gas N_2O, also known as "laughing gas," and modern farming techniques consume a great deal of energy.

At the same time, the "bio" label would be absurd if the fuel came from soy plantations, for instance, that required clearance of a tropical rainforest in Brazil. Biological catastrophes are often linked with CO_2, carbonaceous pollutants and dioxins, as well as pesticides whose usage has long been prohibited in Europe. Scientists from Empa have calculated that bioethanol from rye and potatoes impact the environment five times more than gasoline; the ratio for rapeseed, American corn and Brazilian soy is as much as 2.5-to-1. Of all the cultivated raw materials studied, only grass and wood fared better than gasoline.

However, the study found that biofuels produced from waste and recycled materials (such as liquid manure, sewage sludge and whey) pollute the environment only half as much as gasoline. They are the true "good" raw materials since they need to be disposed of rather than cultivated. Also, a good deal of polluting emissions from existing disposal processes disappear. Although the study suggests that all waste materials should be utilized like this, together they could still only cover a small percentage of fuel consumption.

Who Cloned My Cat? Fun Adventures in Biotechnology by R. Renneberg
Copyright © 2011 by Pan Stanford Publishing Pte Ltd
www.panstanford.com
978-981-4267-65-6

Better results could be achieved by using not only sugar and starch but also cellulose. In order to break down this giant molecule though, new enzymes and microbes are necessary. Biotech can help (see Chap. 76, *Xylophagy in My Bookcase*, p. 167). This could also solve the pervasive problem of land clearance, providing further ecological benefits.

The purpose of the study in Switzerland was to find a proper way of regulating biofuels. Environmental impacts aside, another issue has come into prominence: energy production versus food production. Professor Ghisalba foresees something even worse: conflict triggered by ever-increasing water shortages. Who will want to use it and for what purpose?

I was a little bothered by all this. Why hadn't it occurred to me that biofuels are only a pseudo-solution? My friend Oreste poked fun at me: "If Mr. Bush suddenly started supporting bioalcohol, *then* you'd have given it some very serious thought, eh?!" That good-humored comment — delivered in his cheerful Swiss-German accent — lingered in my ears for the rest of the day!

Read more on this subject in Chap. 69, *Tanking Up with Corn*, p. 151.

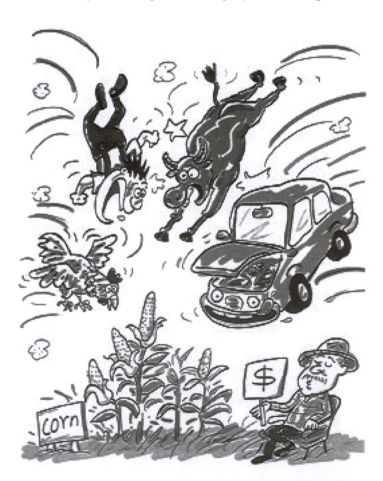

Chapter 80

Microbesoft?

"I can no longer, so to speak, hold my chemical water, and I must tell you that I can make urea without needing a kidney — from a man or a dog," wrote the German chemist Friedrich Wöhler (1800–1882) to his colleague Berzelius in 1828. He had managed to synthesize an organic substance, urea, from inorganic matter, ammonium cyanate. It was revolutionary!

Evidently, gene-mapping guru Craig Venter could also no longer "hold his genetically engineered water" (see Chap. 77, *DNA Gunshots into the Sea*, p. 169). Once again, he has managed to shock his beloved public with wide-ranging patent registrations of a synthetic bacterium. Is it really possible to put a chromosome together gene by gene according to a blueprint and pop it into an empty bacterial cell membrane? Venter is confident that "it" can live.

Mycoplasma genitalium, a harmless urinary tract bacterium, was chosen. It has a very tiny genome, only one tenth that of the genetic engineers' pet, *Escherichia coli*. Venter says, with tremendous humility, "I think one should think of the movie *Superman*. My goal is to save the world." It is his intention, you see, that his patented *Mycobacterium laboratorium* will break down carbon dioxide and produce hydrogen like an energy generator.

Venter brushes off the justifiable scepticism, pointing out that synthetic biology is a very young discipline with only a few of real masters. Master Venter has even said that he doesn't have any knowledge about bacteria — and that is precisely why (!) he has dared to try.

The drum roll came on May 31, 2007, as the patent for *Mycoplasma laboratorium* was granted to the Craig Venter Institute. The synthetic bacterium contains 101 genes fewer than the natural variety. Yet it is still uncertain as to whether it can be successfully manufactured.

A representative of ETC Group, a Canadian organization that monitors technology, raised the alarm. They claimed that the patent was simply an attempt to dominate the market in synthetic biology. Indeed, Venter's patent covers all 381 genes of *Mycoplasma laboratorium* as well as all organisms that will be synthesized

Who Cloned My Cat? Fun Adventures in Biotechnology by R. Renneberg
Copyright © 2011 by Pan Stanford Publishing Pte Ltd
www.panstanford.com
978-981-4267-65-6

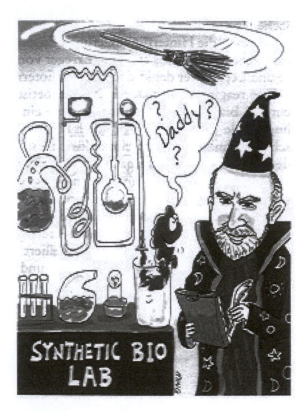

based on this basic genome. In addition, it covers all the variations of the wild-type bacterium that do without at least 55 of the 101 nonessential genes. While there are over 100 types of *Mycoplasma* bacteria, the modified variations of related forms would be protected by the patent as well — a monopoly on knowledge that's very tough for competing scientists. The antics of the Bill Gates empire spring to mind. Perhaps Venter should rename his company *Microbesoft*?

The creation of the synthetic bacterium came with awkward facts: synthetic life forms were brought in through the back door without any discussion. The tuberculosis and leprosy bacteria, incidentally, also belong to the *Mycoplasma* genus. And who hasn't wondered about the potential for bioterrorism?

So, how has the academic synthetic biology community reacted? Well, rather clumsily — a regular sorcerer's apprentice! In 2008, specialists in the field gathered at the Swiss Federal Institute of Technology Zurich (ETH) for their Third International Congress. By their estimation: "…we will have to deal with an explosive mixture of powerful corporations, patent monopolies and messiah complexes. No wonder there's more concern than hope." The Congress also made a lame appeal to governments "to regulate and control the problem."

"Back now, broom, into the closet! Be thou as thou wert before!" (Johann Wolfgang von Goethe's *The Sorcerer's Apprentice*).

Alas, the command didn't come from the sorcerer himself. It's Craig Venter again!

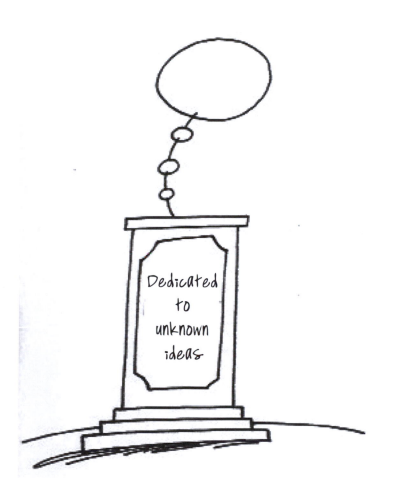